An Extra-Ordinary Guide to Childbirth Preparation

PAM ENGLAND, C.N.N., M.A.
& ROB HOROWITZ, PH.D.

SOUVENIR PRESS

Copyright © 1998 by Pam England & Rob Horowitz
Artwork © 1998 by Pam England
Calligraphy © 1998 by Diana Stetson

First published in the USA by Partera Press

First published in Great Britain in 2007 by Souvenir Press Ltd
43 Great Russell Street, London WC1B 3PD

Reprinted 2011

The right of Pam England and Rob Horowitz to be identified as the authors of this work has been asserted by them in accordance with the Copyright, Designs and Patents Act, 1988

ISBN 13: 9780285637870

Typeset by M Rules in AGaramond
Printed and bound in Great Britain by
CPI Antony Rowe, Chippenham, Wiltshire

CONTENTS

SECTION VII: GESTATING PARENTHOOD

*To Sky and Luc
who taught us about
birthing from within,
and were infinitely patient during
the long labour of writing this book.
And to the mystery
and power
of birth.*

ACKNOWLEDGEMENTS

The development of Birthing From Within was made possible by hundreds of childbirth class students who generously and courageously participated in my eccentric teaching experiments, and gave honest feedback. I (P. E.) also want to thank my midwifery and counselling clients, and the doulas who trained with me, for deepening my understanding and practice of prenatal-birth psychology. The trust and confidence of all these people, too numerous to mention, inspired me through my long years of gestation as a professional.

Those familiar with Zen practice will recognize its influence throughout this book. I want to express my gratitude for Zen training which continues to guide me towards embracing each unfolding moment. I would like to offer heartfelt thanks to my first Zen teacher, Seiju.

One of the last, and most blessed, arrivals as our book neared completion, was our talented book designer, Linda Mae Tratechaud. Linda enthusiastically poured her energy, intelligence, and creativity into this project while she herself prepared for her third birth from within.

A NOTE ABOUT THE STORIES AND BIRTH ART

The colourful birth stories and art that illustrate this book came from the hearts and hands of pregnant mothers and fathers. Great care was taken to make accurate reproductions of original art work. I'm grateful to my clients and research participants for granting permission to publish their art work and stories. With a few permitted exceptions, names and identifying characteristics have been changed to protect confidentiality. (All other pen and ink illustrations were drawn by me, Pam England.)

PHOTOGRAPH AND ART CREDITS

Grateful acknowledgement is made to the following photographers and artists for permission to reproduce their work: Lyn Jones: Photos on pages 14, 17, 63; Meinrad Craighead: BIRTH, 1982 © on page 100, VESSEL, 1983 © on page 99; Judy Chicago: SMOCKED FIGURE 1984 © Needlework by Mary Ewanowski, Chico, CA, on page 64, THE CROWNING, 1985 © Needlework by Susan MacMillan, Janis Wicks, Maggie Eoyang, and Jeanette Russell on page 103; Leah Lee: PAISLEY WOMAN © on page 95, CIRCLE OF LIFE © page 97, and VESSEL 1974 © on page 98; Judy Rominger: PUERTA DE LUNA, © 1989, page 101.

*

We gratefully acknowledge the following for their generous permission to quote from their publications:
     Excerpts from MAMATOTO: A CELEBRATION OF BIRTH by Carroll Dunham and the Body Shop Team. Published by The Penguin Group, reproduced with the permission of The Body Shop International PLC © 1991. The Body Shop International PLC, 1991. All rights reserved.; Permission kindly granted by Norma Bradley Allen to reprint from THE QUILTERS: WOMEN & DOMESTIC ART by Patricia Cooper and Norma Bradley Allen, Copyright © 1978; Permission granted by Paulus Berensohn to use excerpt from FINDING YOUR WAY WITH CLAY by Paulus Berensohn, Copyright © 1972; "Introduction" by Ram Dass, from WHO DIES by Stephen Levine. Copyright © 1982 by Stephen Levine. Used by permission of Doubleday, a division of Bantam Doubleday Dell Publishing Group, Inc.; From THE TRANSITION TO PARENT-HOOD: HOW A FIRST CHILD CHANGES A MARRIAGE by Jay Belsky, Ph.D. and John Kelly. Copyright © 1994 by Jay Belsky, Ph.D. and John Kelly. Used by permission of Delacorte Press, a division of Bantam Doubleday Dell Publishing Group, Inc.; Permission is granted by Doubleday, a division of Bantam Doubleday Dell Publishing Group, Inc. to reproduce excerpts from THE FOXFIRE BOOK by Eliot Wigginton, Editor © 1968; Permission is granted by Bantam Books to quote Corita Kent and Jan Stewart from LEARNING BY HEART: TEACHINGS TO FREE THE CREATIVE SPIRIT, © 1992; Excerpt used as chapter opener from WOMAN AND NATURE: THE ROARING INSIDE HER by Susan Griffin.

Copyright © 1978 by Susan Griffin. Reprinted by permission of HarperCollins Publishers, Inc.; Excerpts from A MIDWIFE'S STORY by Penny Armstrong. Published by Arbor House © 1986. Reprinted with permission from the Martell Agency; Extracts from Judy Graham's article, "A Place to Breathe" is reproduced by kind permission of NURSING TIMES where this article was first published on 20 November 1985; Reprinted from THE HEART OF UNDER-STANDING: COMMENTARIES ON THE PRAJÑAPARAMITA HEART SUTRA (1988) by Thich Nhat Hanh with permission of Parallax Press, Berkeley, California; Excerpts from audiotape "The freedom of No Escape Satsang with Gangaji" given on July 6, 1995. Permission to reproduce granted by Satsang Foundation & Press, 4855 Riverbend Rd. Boulder Co 80301; Reprinted with permission of Sterling Publishing Co., Inc., 387 Park Ave. S., NY, NY 10016 from THE HEALING ART OF TAI CHI: BECOMING ONE WITH NATURE, by Martin Lee, Emily Lee, Melinda Lee, and Joyce Lee, © 1996 by Martin Lee, Emily Lee, Melinda Lee, and Joyce Lee; Excerpts from THE BIRTH PROJECT by Judy Chicago published by Doubleday Anchor Press Copyright © 1985 by Judy Chicago. Reproduced with permission from Through The Flower; Copyright © 1996 by Susan Diamond from HARD LABOR by Susan Diamond. Reprinted by permission of Tom Doherty Associates, Inc.

INTRODUCTION

Gayle Peterson, PhD, author of the groundbreaking *Birthing Normally*, and *An Easier Childbirth*, was an original developer of the Holistic Prenatal Care model which I studied in the early 1980's. Gayle's stimulating and inspirational ideas profoundly influenced the development of my own approach to prenatal preparation.

WHY BIRTHING FROM WITHIN IS AN EXTRA-ORDINARY APPROACH TO CHILDBIRTH PREPARATION

Several fundamental differences make the Birthing from Within approach more than just another childbirth education method. As you'll see, in many ways these classes stand alone.

When I began exploring the possibility of creating a multi-sensory, holistic approach to childbirth education, I had a vision: parents learning through interactive, creative participation, in a spirit of fun and curiosity.

I believed that women already "knew" a lot (whether they knew it or not). So, I developed processes to help them discover and validate their own knowledge, rather than directing a stream of information at them.

Too many classes and books teach new mothers about birth from the "outside," in other words, how it is perceived and managed by professionals. But no mother in the heat of labour is experiencing "stages" or depending on her knowledge of anatomy and physiology to guide her. This kind of knowledge is fascinating, but irrelevant to a mother white-knuckling through a contraction.

The Birthing From Within approach prepares a mother for *birthing from within*. She needs insight about what labour and birth will be like from *her* perspective, and preparation to be in labour and

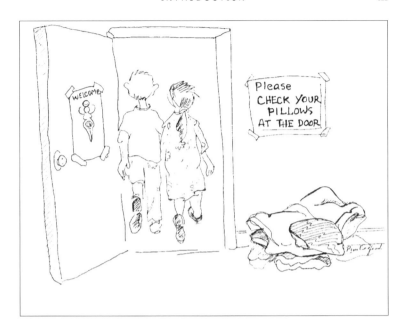

give birth as a mother, not as a trained para-professional. The Birthing From Within classes offer guidance through the emotional, spiritual, psychic and social mists which shroud birthing from within.

The Birthing From Within approach was created and refined over eight years, and continues to evolve. For several years my childbirth classes were known as The Art of Birthing classes. Since the publication of this book, however, they have become Birthing From Within classes. This change reflects more completely the overall philosophy and focus of my teaching approach.

I began with an idea of where I wanted to go, but without a map to get there. I began slowly, one step at a time, but not every step was in the right direction. During many classes I felt like I had walked over a cliff or stumbled into quicksand!

Birthing From Within is a dynamic, organic educational process. Because it is not a crystallized method, there is no predetermined syllabus or curriculum. Feedback from parents not only determines what will be emphasized during their *own* classes, but also refines the process for parents in subsequent classes.

*

Parents often are asked to bring pillows to other childbirth classes for the purpose of lying comfortably on floor mats practising relaxation techniques. My first small step on the journey was to banish comfy pillows from the teaching room. The medium is the message: I wanted parents to understand that not only was labour hard *work*, but it wasn't something they should do lying down. I specifically wanted to avoid strengthening cultural images of labouring women lying in a hospital bed practising stylized relaxation techniques.

In our classes we explore personal and cultural beliefs about labour pain. Parents learn how these beliefs affect their experience of, and ability to cope with, pain. We devote significant time to practising the mindful pain coping techniques described in Section Six. At the same time, there remains an open-mindedness to the compassionate use of pain medications.

*

The usual focus of childbirth education is limited to what happens in labour. But parents are hungry for other kinds of information. They want to know what to do *after* the baby is born. I realized that childbirth preparation should also be parent preparation.

So my next step was to teach expectant parents baby care basics, such as how to swaddle, soothe and bathe their newborn, teach their baby to sleep, and get nursing off to a good start. We often sing lullabies (sometimes with kazoo accompaniment by the parents). Mothers and fathers love learning how to care for their newborn. They tell me it boosts their confidence and makes them even more eager for their baby to arrive.

*

I consider the introduction of making birth art to be my most significant innovation in teaching childbirth classes. At first I worried that asking parents to draw, paint or sculpt would result in a parade of drop-outs. But to my amazement, making birth art became the favourite activity for many of the parents in my classes.

Even for the timid and inexperienced, the art-making process is fun and relaxing. It's a time for parents to reflect on what they know, need, want, fear, and remember. Talking about their art prompts important questions and initiates lively discussions. Thus, in a reversal of the usual class structure, the class which is typically passive

Another important distinction between Birthing From Within classes and the majority of other classes, is their location and ambience. The setting for classes sends a powerful meta-message to the unconscious of new parents. That's why right from the start, I felt it was important to teach Birthing From Within classes in a home-like setting, unaffiliated with any medical institution.

When I began, I taught classes out of my home. As their popularity grew, I moved the Art of Birthing Center into a little house converted into a cozy office space. Care was taken to choose warm, earth-tone colours; pretty lace curtains were hung. The walls are decorated with the colourful birth art made by parents taking classes. Flowers, a friendly tea hutch and gently trickling water fountain welcome visitors.

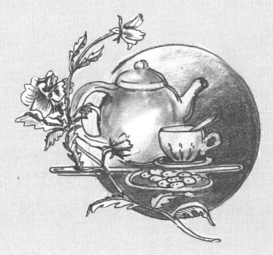

The environment is an expression of the Birthing From Within philosophy and provides a backdrop for what unfolds during the classes. A relaxed, informal setting puts people at ease, normalizes having a baby, and energizes class interaction. This more active involvement in childbirth *preparation* sets the stage for more active involvement in *childbirth*.

becomes "active," and offers inspiration and direction to the teacher. This move to a more symmetrical learning relationship is another part of what makes Birthing From Within extra-ordinary.

My work with pregnant women has shown me that giving creative expression to secret hopes and dark fears is a vital part of childbirth preparation. Daring to express oneself through painting, sculpting or poetry is a way a mother (or father) boldly says, "I made this, it's about what I know, what I feel as a mother (or father). This is me." This self expression, and the acknowledgment and validation given by the group, infuses mothers with new confidence and strength.

*

Another subtle difference (between Birthing From Within classes and institutional classes) that parents should be aware of: classes taught in and by an institution can't help but send the message "You are now on our turf. Listen, and we'll tell you how *we'll* deliver your baby when you come here." It's understandable that teachers will be familiar with, support, even defend the policies and procedures of the institution that hired them. The indirect hypnotic messages sent by both the ambience and content in an institutional classroom suggest what your role in birth is likely to be (i.e., that of a passive patient).

PHILOSOPHICAL ASSUMPTIONS AND GUIDING PRINCIPLES OF BIRTHING FROM WITHIN CHILDBIRTH CLASSES

1. Childbirth is a profound rite of passage, not a medical event (even when medical care is part of the birth).
2. The essence of childbirth preparation is self-discovery, not assimilating obstetric information.
3. The teacher is "midwife" to the parents' discovery process, not the expert from whom wisdom flows.
4. Childbirth preparation is a continually evolving process (for parents and teachers), not a static structure of techniques and knowledge.
5. Parents' individual needs and differences determine class content.
6. Active, creative self-expression is critical to childbirth preparation.

7. The purpose of childbirth preparation is to prepare mothers to give birth-in-awareness, not to achieve a specific birth outcome.

8. Pregnancy and birth outcome are influenced by a variety of factors, but can't be *controlled* by planning.

9. In order to help parents mobilize their coping resources, it is critical for childbirth classes to acknowledge that unexpected, unwelcome events may happen during labour.

10. Parents deserve support for any birth option which might be right for them (whether it be drugs, technology, home birth, or bottle-feeding).

11. Pain is an inevitable part of childbirth, yet much can be done to ease *suffering*.

12. Pain coping techniques work best when integrated into daily life, rather than "dusted off" for labour.

13. Fathers help best as birth guardians or loving partners, not as coaches; *they* also need support.

14. For parents, pregnancy, birth, and postpartum is a time of continuous learning and adjustment; holistic support and education should be available throughout that period.

15. Childbirth preparation is also parent preparation.

THE FOOTBATH RITUAL: AN EXAMPLE OF OUR NON-TRADITIONAL APPROACH

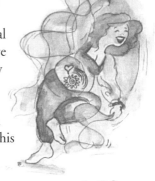

To give you a feel for the non-traditional Birthing From Within exercises, I've included a description of a new favourite, The Footbath Ritual.

One day a friend gave me a package of colourful paper plates decorated with a pregnant woman and the message, "This Woman Deserves A Party." I loved these plates and taped one of them to a wall at the Art of Birthing Center.

Pregnant women really *do* deserve a party, to celebrate what their bodies have done and are about to do. Don't you agree? I realized that the Birthing From Within classes should do even more to recognize birth as a rite of passage.

At the next childbirth class, I talked to all the fathers secretly. I invited each to participate in a rite of passage for his partner to help her make the uncharted journey into Labourland. I told each father to bring four things to the next (and last) class: a basin for a foot bath, a towel, massage oil and a blessing, wish, prayer or poem for her journey. All the fathers liked the idea and agreed to do it. I was touched, and a bit surprised, by their enthusiasm.

With a half-hour remaining in the last class, I asked the fathers to follow me to another room. Their first task was to claim a favourite chair or space at the Center for the surprise footbath.

Then we all crowded into the kitchen where they filled their basins with warm water. I gave each a bowl of flowers, rose petals and lavender to float in the water. The dads poured their partners a cup of herbal pregnancy tea.

I gave one last instruction. I suggested they use this footbath as another (blissful) opportunity to practise the mindful pain-coping techniques learned in earlier classes (e.g., breath awareness, non-focused awareness, and touch-relaxation).

Now they were ready for their mission …

*

Moments later, the Center was humming with quiet talk, laughter and music. The fragrance of flowers and oils hung in the air. Mothers, eyes closed and feet covered with colourful petals, oozed relaxed contentment. During the foot massage, the fathers had a chance to bring together nurturance and tenderness while guiding their partners through labour support techniques they had learned in class.

Afterwards the group reassembled, and I was struck by how connected and mellow everyone seemed. It occurred to me that the footbath ritual might be the most lasting memory to come from our classes. I sensed that for some couples, this intimate moment would be a wellspring for tender touching and communication during their birth, and even beyond. By the end of the evening I knew the footbath "experiment" was an innovation worth keeping.

BIRTHING FROM WITHIN CHILDBIRTH CLASSES ARE NOT A STATIC COLLECTION OF TECHNIQUES.

This approach is an on-going exploration utilizing any of the following exercises and activities ... and new ones are still being developed!

- Making Birth Art
- Journaling and Poetry Reading
- Exploring Assumptions About Pain
- Extensive Training in Pain Coping Techniques
- Tracking and Taming Birth Tigers
- Birth and Placenta Customs: An Anthro-Exploration
- Telling Family Birth Stories and Traditions
- A Special Class for Fathers and Birth Companions
- Role Playing
- A Footbath Ritual
- Coyote Howling
- Singing Lullabies
- Unfoldment Process (experiencing birth from the baby's perspective)
- Babyproofing Your Marriage

*

HOW TO GET THE MOST FROM THIS BOOK

The profound mystery and spirituality of birth can never be understood with the mind; they are known through the heart. It is this knowing from the heart which is critical for women in preparing for their rite of passage. Birthing From Within's multi-sensory approach has evolved to help women and their partners make that journey in awareness, and with heightened confidence.

This approach is not a theory being offered for testing in the "real world;" it's a presentation of what actually has worked for me with parents in childbirth education. These exercises have challenged and intrigued countless mothers and fathers, and have often been the key to insights which would have remained undiscovered in a typical childbirth class.

Birthing From Within is not a script or a rigid method. Every parent or professional who reads this book should choose and adapt what matches their personality and their needs. You can get a lot out of this book simply by reading and reflection. But the greatest rewards are likely if you actually *practise* the exercises and techniques. Approach each one with an open-ended curiosity rather than with a specific goal in mind (you can approach the unknown experience of labour in the same way).

I recommend you keep a spiral notebook, an easy-flowing pen, and coloured pencils or markers handy. You can record questions, insights, imagery or dreams that come up while reading or doing the exercises. (Beware: stay away from pretty journals! They might inhibit you from being spontaneous, messy, wild and free.)

You will probably want to have a few art supplies on hand in case you have a burst of creative energy—there is a list on page 48.

You can work alone. However, sharing these exercises in a small group may enhance your insight, understanding, and empathy while helping you connect with other parents.

MY JOURNEY: PAM

The joy, passion, and pain I felt as a nurse, midwife, mother and pre-natal-birth therapist inspired the creation of Birthing From Within. I want to share with you, the reader, where the roots of this book lie.

*

I cried when I saw my first birth in nursing school (1973). I had created a mental picture of women as strong and primal in labour, and viewed the process as sacred, natural, and at the same time, ordinary. I cried, though, not because it was such a miracle, but because it was so violent.

The mother was alone (because her husband was told to wait in the waiting room); she lay medicated and exhausted in a narrow bed, constrained by the foetal monitor. Just as she was ready to push, her doctor insisted on spinal anaesthesia, which completely immobilized her from the waist down. Two nurses dragged her in a sheet from her bed to a cart. She was wheeled from her labour cubicle back to the surgical stainless steel delivery room, where she was pulled from the cart to the delivery table. Nurses lifted her floppy, numb legs into stirrups, fully exposing her genitals. Hospital staff in masks, booties, and gloves were rushing around. One nurse shaved the mother's pubic area and washed her denuded perineum with cold betadine solution, while another aimed the glaring surgical light hanging from the ceiling. The doctor, fully gowned, gloved and masked entered and perfunctorily cut her episiotomy, applied forceps to her baby's head, and pulled him out.

When she spontaneously reached for her newborn, the nurses frantically yelled, "Don't touch him!" The worried mother's arms recoiled as she asked, "Why not? What's wrong?," only to learn, "The drapes are sterile. Keep your hands under the drapes." And the doctor handed her baby to the nurse.

The child she had dreamed about for months was taken to the far end of the delivery room, out of reach, even out of sight. The distraught mother could hear him screaming as his feet were needlessly and repeatedly slapped – until the nurses and doctor were satisfied that his lungs were "healthy."

As a student-nurse, I often found myself standing out in the hall by the labour and delivery rooms, bewildered and disturbed. Even though I wasn't aware of home births and midwives at the time, I knew women did not have to give birth *this* way.

Shortly after, I learned about midwifery. Once I began my midwifery training at the Frontier Nursing Service in Hyden, Kentucky (1977), I knew I had come home. Everything I learned and did made sense to me. During the next five years, I practiced midwifery in the hospital and a birth centre, and also attended women at home.

*

I was elated when I then became pregnant. I had every confidence that the birth of my child would be like those of the women in my family, and the majority of women I had been midwife to: strong and powerful, in a peaceful, familiar home setting.

Although my pregnancy was medically normal, I felt an undercurrent of tension and fear with which I did not know how to deal. I had concerns about what kind of mother I would be. I was planning a home birth, and worried about something going wrong which would require transfer to a hospital where I would face losing control of my birth, or having a Caesarean.

But, at the time, I believed that worrying or talking about my fears could make them happen, and that "positive thinking" would make everything perfect. And because my pregnancy was medically normal, I was given superficial reassurance when I brought up my fears or nightmares. I was ready to accept such reassurance because I assumed that as a nurse-midwife, I already knew everything I needed to know about giving birth.

Weeks later, in the midst of my long and difficult labour, I realized nothing I had learned as a nurse-midwife was helping me, but it was too late to learn what I really needed to know about giving birth as a mother.

Finally, strapped to an operating table, anaesthetized and draped, I gave birth to my son, Sky, by Caesarean. As I was being sewn up, I mused over the painful irony, that I, the person in my family who knew the most about birth, was the first to have a Caesarean. "How did this happen?," I wondered. "Was there something I needed to know that I didn't learn as a midwife?"

*

Through soul-searching
and listening more deeply
to the women I was working with,
I finally understood that women
have to prepare for birth
in their heart and soul,
not their head.
And that giving birth is something a woman does
in her body,
not in her head.

*

I came to realize, as a mother and a midwife, how even a well-meaning focus on potential birth problems and birth technology throughout pregnancy distracts the mother-to-be from the more vital task of *inner* preparation. The choices in birth technology available to women today are so mind-boggling that in trying to understand the complex world of obstetrics, many lose faith in their own ability to birth. Thus, many women cannot give birth, and in the end must rely on the very technology that mystified them in the first place.

*

During my second pregnancy, I knew my greatest task was to "forget" all I had learned as a nurse-midwife so that I could "remember" my instincts. I had to learn how to simply be a mother, not a patient or a pregnant-medical-professional.

I learned to sit quietly with my heartfelt questions and deepest fears as well as actively making birth art, contemplating birth stories and customs, keeping a journal, and finally, learning to embrace the unknowable and unplannable nature of birth.

I'll always believe that this work I did before, and during, my second pregnancy made all the difference. Luc was born quickly and peacefully at home. That birth restored a balance to my understanding of what birth could be, as well as how to prepare for it.

*

As a prenatal-birth therapist and childbirth educator, I try to help women develop a calm, curious and receptive state of mind rather than just filling their heads with seemingly useful knowledge. The child of my personal and professional life, The Art of Birthing evolved into the holistic approach which I share in this book.

*

As you've already noticed, there are two authors of this book, although the text is written in the first person. This is because I, Pam, created and work with this method as a midwife and teacher, and wrote the original draft of this book. The clarity of thought and simple grace of language in the book, however, are largely a credit to my co-author, Rob Horowitz, whose original degree was in English literature. He spent countless hours in discussion, editing, and rewriting. Rob also contributed his perspectives as a psychologist, family systems expert, husband and father, as well as his unique sense of humour. He has been an enthusiastic and unflagging source of encouragement in my development of both the Birthing From Within approach and this book.

MY JOURNEY: ROB

Reflecting back seven years to the months before our son, Luc, was born, I'm amazed, and a bit humbled, by how profoundly ignorant I was about birth. The six years that I spent with Pam working on our book have enlightened and excited me about birth, which I now *feel* as part of the core of human experience. This awareness has deepened my work as a therapist.

Pam's vision, passion, and commitment to helping women have fuelled our gruelling, exhilarating creative journey together. She was *determined* to light a path by which pregnant women could regain their emotional, psychological, and spiritual birthright. During this process, I came to appreciate the drama unfolding within each new parent and each new couple, as well as how our society is struggling to re-humanize birth. I caught "birth fever" from Pam, and for that I'm grateful.

Pam England & Rob Horowitz
July 17, 1997
Albuquerque, New Mexico

SECTION I

Beginning Your Journey

.

1

Finding Your Question

Understanding birth technology shouldn't lull you into
thinking you understand *birth*. The profound mystery and
spirituality of birth can never be understood with the mind,
they are known through the heart. A good place to begin
preparing is with your heart's burning question.

A journalism student once asked me, "If there is one thing a woman
should know before going into labour, what would you say it would
be?"

I mulled this question over for a while. In the past, women knew
what had to be done, and with a mixture of fear, power and surrender—they did it. Giving birth was part of their normal lives. Only
now are women drawn off course by exotic (yet peripheral) choices:
which books to read … and what to believe; which tests to accept or
decline; where to give birth and … with whom; to flee from pain …
or not; and finally, which interventions, if any, would be right for
them.

After contemplating the journalist's question, I finally responded,
"For each woman, the most important thing she needs to know will
be different. I would encourage a mother to ask herself, 'What is it I
need to know to give birth?' Her answer must be found within, not
given to her by an expert. Each mother needs to find her personal,
heartfelt question."

The journalist wasn't sure she understood what I meant, so I asked
her, "When you were expecting, what was it you needed to know to
give birth?"

She thought a moment, and smiled as she remembered, "My question was 'Am I strong enough to give birth?' That's what I worried
about, that's what I had to look into before I felt ready to give
birth … and I did use that question to help me prepare mentally."

Mothers wonder things like:

- "What kind of mother will I be?"
- "Can I ask for help if I need it?"
- "Can I trust my body and my judgement?"
- "What will people think of me if … ?"
- "Who gives birth?"

*

Knowing your personal question is central to birth preparation. Whatever your question is, leave no stone unturned: ask your question often and look at it from every angle until your conscious mind is exhausted, and your heart is receptive to answers.

Don't limit yourself to a superficial question like, "What should I expect …?" If someone else can answer your question—you're not going deep enough. The answer will not come through intellectual pursuit; nor will you find it in a book (books can tell you about birth, but not about *you*).

Sometimes true understanding comes in a dream, when you're gazing into a fire, writing in your journal, after a good cry, or when you finally give up! Be patient: sometimes the answer doesn't surface until the throes of labour!

PREGNANT WOMEN FACE A DILEMMA:

Do they take the risk of knowing too much, or of knowing too little?

WHAT DO WOMEN NEED TO KNOW TO GIVE BIRTH TO DAY?

Contemporary women who are birthing in a hospital need two kinds of knowing. The first, and most basic, is *primordial knowing*, that innate capability which modern women have but must rediscover (and trust). The second kind is *modern knowing*: being savvy about the medical and hospital culture and how to give birth within it. Birthing from within requires both these kinds of knowing.

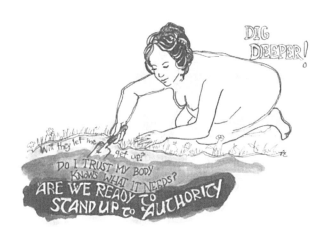

Chapter 2

Emptying Your Mind

The mind of the beginner is empty, free of the habits of the expert, ready to accept, to doubt, and open to all the possibilities.

RICHARD BAKER FROM INTRODUCTION TO *ZEN MIND, BEGINNER'S MIND* BY SHUNRYO SUZUKI

In one sense, you've been in childbirth classes since you were a toddler. The world you were born into is the blueprint for your thought patterns and assumptions about what being human means. As a girl playing house, you internalized your culture's messages about motherhood.

So, long before you discovered you were pregnant, your capacity to experience pregnancy and birth had already been constricted by years of "schooling." This process is both seamless and invisible.

To the degree cultural assumptions go unnoticed or unquestioned, you are limited by them. Not so long ago, pregnant women were afraid to hang their laundry, believing that raising their arms above their head would cause the cord to wrap around the baby's neck. In every phase of history, including our own, practices based on erroneous assumptions are the norm.

The more aware you are of what has been your unconscious or conditioned learning, the more you can actually see what *is*, and embrace whatever comes up in your pregnancy and birth. Question assumptions you've accepted as "true." *True* understanding springs from an open, curious mind, and can be achieved only after the cultural blinders of conditioned learning have been removed.

Much as a Zen practitioner works years to eliminate internal "chatter" to be in the moment, you, as a mother, must learn to put aside

TRY THIS:

(THIS REALLY DOES TAKE PRACTISE!)

Sit quietly. Sit straight up so you can breathe easily, feel energized and alert. Notice how thoughts and ideas naturally come and go, floating freely in the mind.

A particular idea or fantasy may dominate your thinking, blocking your flow of awareness. Just notice, without judgement, when this happens, and follow the thought-image to its source. You can do this by gently questioning and exploring all aspects of your thought-image until finally you reach the empty, open place of now-knowing.

All customs, beliefs and assumptions are just "ideas," yours or somebody else's. If you look deeply into ideas, you will find emptiness. If your mind becomes attached to a certain point of view, gently remind yourself, "This is just my idea."

preconceived notions and judgements to *be*–in–birth. Your quest, like that of the Zen student, is to clear the clouding layer of thought between you and your experience.

In birth preparation, your first task is to empty your mind of expectations and judgements that narrow the possibilities for coping with pain, surprises and the hard work of labour. Being "empty" will allow you to receive, moment-by moment, the messages conveyed by your body, mind and heart.

A genuine emptying of the mind requires a commitment to sustained attention. Paying attention creates opportunities for a powerful birth in awareness, be it natural or not. Just as an embracing of life includes, inevitably, an embracing of death, there will be some women for whom an embracing of birth must include their experience of a difficult birth.

Just before women give birth, many experience the primitive "nesting" instinct: an intense surge of energy to clean and prepare the home for the imminent arrival of the new baby. There is also a psychological nesting to be done throughout pregnancy: a "housecleaning" of the mind.

Something which comes out of nothingness is naturalness,
For a plant or stone to be natural is no problem.
But for us there is some problem …
To be natural is something which we must work on.

SHUNRYO SUZUKI, ZEN MASTER, *ZEN MIND, BEGINNER'S MIND*

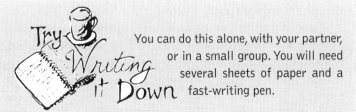

You can do this alone, with your partner, or in a small group. You will need several sheets of paper and a fast-writing pen.

For ten to fifteen minutes

Write as fast as you can anything and everything
you assume to be true about pregnancy, labour,
birth and being a mother.
Write your birth legacy:
family/religious/cultural beliefs, images, fears,
traditions, unforgettable birth stories, and
old wives' tales.
Go!

Read aloud what you wrote. Consider having someone else read it aloud so you can listen with your whole body-mind to the words and imagery you wrote.

What is the overall feeling in what you wrote? What beliefs and assumptions are contained in it? Be curious!

Where did these assumptions come from in the first place? (a moment of reverie? a family tradition or myth? your own experience or fears? a movie, a friend, or a prophet-of-doom who stood behind you in the grocery checkout?)

How does keeping this idea, fear, or belief, work for you?

If this idea evaporated, who would you be? What would you do differently?

Interestingly, you don't have to find an "answer." Continually asking and asking your questions brings deeper understanding and opens the mind to greater possibilities.

Chapter 3

Worry Is the Work of Pregnancy

Our study group in Albuquerque resisted when Dr. Lewis Mehl, a psychologist who specializes in childbirth-related issues, said, "Worry *is* the work of pregnancy." We were all holding on to the notion that women who appear relaxed, confident and together, birth normally.

We were intrigued by his story about a childbirth class in Georgia. There were six couples in that class. One of the couples was particularly concerned about how to avoid a Caesarean birth. Every week, they stretched the patience of their childbirth teacher with questions. Later, at the group's postpartum reunion, everyone was amazed that the couple who had worried so much about a Caesarean birthed normally, while the five couples who had sat quietly all had Caesareans!

In the years to follow, my midwifery practice taught me that for some women, worry *is* the work of pregnancy. In fact, an overconfident first-time mum who thinks she has it all figured out, worries me. I worry she will not be truly prepared for what awaits her.

Women all over the world worry about pain, the health of their baby, and of dying in labour. Western mothers have additional worries: whether their own doctor or midwife will be on call when they're in labour, avoiding unnecessary interventions, separation from their newborn and the cost of medical care.

WORRYING EFFECTIVELY

Hannah, a second-time mum, wanted to have a simple, natural birth experience after having had a highly medicalized birth. Her worry that this birth would be another painful disappointment clouded her pregnancy. She remained immobilized and ambivalent into her eighth month.

She longed to hear me say that everything would be all right. Even though her problems were not likely to recur, I resisted the socially expected, "Don't worry" response. Empty reassurance might have supported her avoidance of the hard, painful work she still needed to do.

Hannah wanted to believe that positive thinking would make this birth work out, yet intuitively, we both knew that more was needed. Instead, I encouraged her to face what she feared. In trying to control her fears, Hannah hadn't been worrying enough!

The first task I gave her was to write down all her secret worries. "Some of your worries may be genuinely trivial," I suggested, "but look closely at the ones you are trying to minimize or ignore. Pay particular attention to worries that create a physical tension in your body."

When Hannah brought her worry-list to our next session, we explored each worry using the following questions:

- What would you do if this worry/fear actually happened?
- What do you imagine your partner (or birth attendant) would do/say?
- What would it mean about you (as a mother) if this happened?
- How have you faced crises in the past?
- What, if anything, can you do to prepare for, or even prevent, what you are worrying about? What's keeping you from doing it?
- If there's nothing you can do to prevent it, how would you like to handle the situation?

Some people believe that exploring fears or worries make them more likely to happen. In fact, worrying *effectively* helped Hannah shift from frozen, fearful images of not being able to cope, to more fluid images containing a variety of coping responses. Weeks later, Hannah gave birth simply and normally to her daughter, Laura, in a hospital birthing room.

TEN COMMON WORRIES

- Not being able to stand the pain
- Not being able to relax
- Feeling rushed, or fear of taking too long
- My pelvis not big enough
- My cervix won't open
- Lack of privacy

- Being judged for making noise
- Being separated from the baby
- Having to fight for my wishes to be respected
- Having intervention and not knowing if it is necessary or what else to do

FEAR OF DYING IN LABOUR

> Every time one of my babies was about to be born, I'd think to myself, "You're going to die! This time you're going to die!" Then it'd come out. Somehow—I don't know how to explain it—but somehow it was like *I* had been born again.
>
> IN THE WORDS OF AN ITALIAN PEASANT
> FROM KATHRYN ALLEN RABUZZI, *MOTHERSELF*

Women the world over worry when facing the daunting task of navigating the unknown journey of labour. The three worries shared among women everywhere are: fear of pain, fear of having an abnormal or dead baby, and fear of dying in labour.

We seldom hear of a mother dying in labour. So learning that some mothers have fleeting fears of dying surprises, and perhaps unnerves us. Interestingly, mothers tell me that when the thought of dying surfaced near the end of labour, they were simply aware of the thought or feeling, perhaps surprised, but not disturbed by it.

Why does this thought of dying come up in a healthy labour, often just before giving birth? The mounting intensity of labour forces complete surrender of our body and will, dissolving our egos, ideas, and familiar sense of self. We're not afraid of dying because there is no "self" left to resist and fear. At that transcendent moment we have become *birth* itself. This is the spiritual birth of woman into mother.

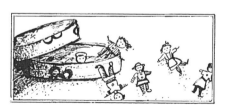

Guatemalan worry dolls: each one takes on a worry of its owner.

Chapter 4

Connecting With Other Women

In the last, most intense hours of labour, I had unexpectedly become mindless, floating in boundless empty space between contractions, unoccupied by any thoughts whatsoever. This timeless bliss was regularly pierced by sharp pain reminding me that my head was still attached to a body! But in between contractions, my mind would simply float away.

Near the end of labour, my ego, mental chatter and birth plans all receded into the activity of birth. My thinking-mind plummeted into an immense silence in which I felt bathed in love and well-being.

It was then, for an unforgettable moment, that I felt a oneness with all mothers who had ever given birth, and to mothers all over the world who were labouring and giving birth with me that night. For a fleeting moment, I saw all of us reaching deep inside for strength to break through the mental and physical limitations which we, as maidens, had assumed to exist.

No longer feeling isolated, I noticed a surge of compassion and vigor. Strange as it may sound, it seemed that my effort was in some way helping others through labour, and their effort was helping me. In giving birth to Sky, I had become a link in the eternal chain of Mothers.

This profound sense of connection with other women was a turning point, not only in my labour but in my understanding as a childbirth teacher.

Your next task then, is to renew and affirm your connection with other women. This chapter revives three traditional ways of doing this: 1) Sharing Birth Stories; 2) Mother Blessings; and 3) Making a Butterfly or Friendship Crib Quilt; Reviving the Quilting Bee.

*

SHARING BIRTH STORIES

Women, traditionally, have turned to other women for advice and sustenance during pregnancy. Sometimes I begin a class by asking couples to recount family birth stories. I ask them to share their mothers', grandmothers' and great-grandmothers' birth stories. These accounts range from inspiring to hilarious—and teach us a great deal. Listen to these stories:

MY GRANDMA MARY'S STORY

My grandmother had only one child, to whom she gave birth in a cold-water flat in Chicago in 1930. When I asked her to tell me her birth story, this is what she said:

> I kept working around the apartment when I was in labour. What else can you do? When I knew that your mother was going to be born soon, I sent someone for the doctor. Doctors came to the house in those days, I didn't know of any midwives.
>
> He must have brought a nurse who was new to this. I remember he told her to "tie some sheets around the legs." And she tied torn strips of sheets around my ankles. I didn't know why she was doing this. I never had a baby before.
>
> The doctor got flustered with the nurse and scolded her, "No! Not around Mary's legs, around the legs of the bed!" I guess the [strips of] sheets were to help me pull on something when I pushed. I don't know what happened then, but before she could get the sheets tied right, your mother was born.

My grandmother laughed to herself when she told me this story. She was gazing downward as though seeing it again for the first time in years.

A few months later, at the time I discovered I was pregnant with my first child, my grandmother died. But her story of my mother's birth is alive in me and preserved in my journal.

FINA'S STORY TOLD BY PAULA

This story was told to our class by Paula, who had grown up in Brazil. Fina, short for Josaphina, was the family maid during Paula's childhood.

Fina had six children born between 1953 and 1964, and liked to tell her birth stories. She told me that she gave birth to her first two by herself, but her mother was with her for the last

When her first two children were born, she lived in a rural area in central Brazil, in the state of Minas Gerais. She worked in the fields ... and went into labour while picking and harvesting, but went right on working because she knew she would have the labour pains anyway, so she might as well work until the water broke. When her water broke, she walked home and gave birth.

The last four were born in the coastal city of Sao Paulo; but she still preferred to labour in complete privacy. Fina believed that giving birth to her children was her business, and she wanted to do it alone. Her husband was not at any of the births. She laboured alone, and pushed alone.

She locked her other kids in their bedroom while she was in hard labour because she didn't want them running outside without supervision.

Her mother stood outside the door, listening for the right moment to walk in and help.

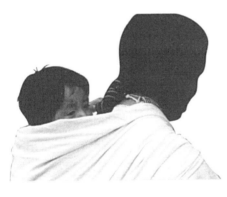

Photo credit: Lyn Jones

MERIA'S STORY

Attended by a midwife, Meria had her three babies at home. She experienced giving birth the first time, lying on her back, as more painful than she had expected. When she became pregnant with her second child, she wrote to her grandmother Meta, asking for advice.

My Grandma Meta's parents were German immigrants. They settled in Grand Rapids, Michigan. They lived on Lowell Avenue for 45 years, in the same house in which their children were born and raised.

She wrote back that she, too, had given birth the first time on her back (in 1919) and found it painful. So, during her second pregnancy, my grandmother asked her midwife for advice. Her midwife told her to "stand up and it would go better."

My grandmother described how in labour she stood and held on to her buffet during contractions and while pushing—and her second birth was much easier and less painful. She sent me this advice in a letter, "Hold on to your buffet."

A buffet is a piece of furniture about four feet high by six feet long, with drawers to hold linen, silver, and dishes. Meria remembered her grandmother's immaculate house and her buffet "polished to a glistening."

It just so happened that during her second pregnancy Meria had a buffet, much like her grandmother's. "A table can be a bit low for a labouring mother to lean on, but, a buffet was just right!"

This is Meria's birth story:

> I was up and about in labour. It was only two hours before the urge to push came. I held onto the buffet and pushed, then walked away and pushed in a squatting position, and finally pushed holding onto my husband … and my baby was born! It was the easiest and least painful of my three births.
>
> During my third birth, the midwife made me lie down to deliver the baby, and it hurt much more.

LESLIE'S MOTHER'S STORY

Nesting often takes the most mundane form as Leslie learned when she talked to her mother:

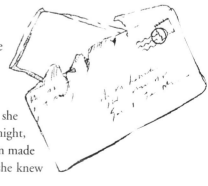

> My mother told me when she realized she was in labour in the middle of the night, she got up and cleaned the house, then made my dad a lunch and supper because she knew

she wouldn't be home the next day. She washed the laundry and ironed my dad's clothes. She didn't want to wake him and worry him during the night.

She cooked breakfast, but he noticed she wasn't eating, and figured out she was in labour. They went to the hospital and the baby, my older brother, was born three hours later.

MOTHERS KNOW SOMETHING OTHER PEOPLE DON'T BUT SOMETIMES THEY DON'T KNOW IT

There are unique things that only experienced mothers can teach pregnant women about birth. However, the majority of women you will encounter will underestimate or devalue their personal experience and wisdom.

The medicalization of birth has left three generations of women spiritually and psychologically wounded. But no matter what her experience in birth was, every mother knows something other people don't know. However, she may not know it. Or she may not realize that her deepest understanding is what you are really interested in. If you want more than a medical report, you have to ask the right questions!

ANCIENT WOMAN, ANCIENT MOTHER

My first encounter with Lucy abruptly changed the direction of my preparation for childbirth. Lucy is on display at the Maxwell Museum of Anthropology at the University of New Mexico in Albuquerque. She is 3 feet, 7 inches tall, a life-like model of an early human who lived 3.6 million years ago in Africa.

When anthropologists found her, they also discovered footprints made by both a large and a small adult, as well as the tracks of a child who walked in the prints of one of the adults.

My awareness shifted from seeing Lucy as an ancient woman to recognizing her as an ancient mother. Sitting with Lucy and painting her picture emptied my modern woman-midwifery mind and made space for a different kind of knowing.

When Lucy was pregnant, she did not know how or when she conceived. She was not preoccupied with how many centimetres her

TRY THESE QUESTIONS:

- What helped you most when you gave birth?
- What was your spiritual experience of giving birth?
- If you could do it over again, what would you do the same?
- Is there anything you would do differently?
- What do you wish you had known beforehand?

If the wise mothers in your life are not available to you, or you don't have someone else you can confide in, I suggest you do try this:

Create a detailed, mental picture of a grandmother, a remembered or imaginary one. Then ask her the questions listed above.

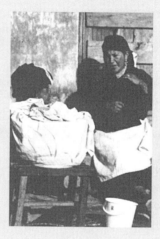

Photo credit: Lyn Jones

uterus was, how many grams of protein she ate, or when her due date was. She lived moment-to-moment, unconsciously responding to her gradually changing patterns in sleep, diet, and movement as her belly grew full.

The day Lucy went into labour, she didn't know how many centimetres she was dilated, whether she was one day early or two weeks late. There was no one who could communicate what she needed to do. She automatically responded to her body's messages; instinctively she knew when to stop eating, when to rest, how to breathe differently or even screech. As her baby was being born, Lucy spontaneously grunted and pushed.

I became absorbed in my fantasy of how Lucy gave birth, and tried to imagine what it might be like to give birth primally, without self-consciousness. For the first time, I understood that if I tried to force, control or give birth in any particular way, to fit a preconceived notion, it would not be "natural."

RENEWING A RITE OF PASSAGE: MOTHER BLESSINGS

In a birth art session, Renata's pastel drawing of *Being Pregnant* (Figure 4.1) beautifully depicts a mother's "incubation" and metamorphosis from maiden to mother, and her initiation into the secret, ancient society of Mothers.

Like many modern women, Renata yearned for other mothers to recognize and guide her spiritual transition into motherhood. While talking about her drawing, she reflected on her recent baby shower, and how disappointing it was for her:

> Everybody was generous and happy, but afterwards I was terribly depressed. There was a huge pile of baby presents, yet not one woman recognized me as a mother. If a baby shower is supposed to get a mother ready it should be something different. It's not just about babies … There was nothing that connected me with other women— but mothers know something that other people don't know—and they should tell us, get us ready.

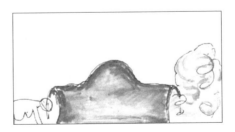

FIGURE 4.1 "It looks like an oven, a cave, or an *horno* (a type of oven used by Pueblo Indians to make bread). You go in there alone … give birth in there … it's more like an incubation [of motherhood] than birth. On the other side you join all the women who have ever done it."
Renata

Our custom of baby showers is a hollow remnant of rituals originally designed to help women prepare for the transformation of self during birth. What had been a mother's sacred rite of passage has become the shallow, trivializing baby shower.

This change mirrors the shift in the medical culture. In recent years, obstetrics has changed its focus from mother-centred care to baby-centred care (throughout prenatal care and during labour).

The movement of medical technology into the foreground of birth has also included the emergence of the doctor, midwife or nurse as the central character in the drama. All too often mothers have been relegated to playing a supporting role (with few, if any, lines); the importance of their emotional and spiritual experience has been eased off stage.

CELEBRATING THE MOTHER

> Celebration is a kind of food we all need in our lives, … each individual brings a special recipe or offering, so that together we make a great feast.
>
> CORITA KENT
> *LEARNING BY HEART*

After a birth in our baby-focused culture we announce: "A baby has been born." In a mother-focused culture like the Ticopia of the Solomon Islands, the birth of child is announced by saying "A mother has given birth."[1] The colourful pastel of birth (Figure 4.2) drawn by a mother of four, beautifully portrays "mother as the centre of attention."

Even though the rituals surrounding birth have changed with the advent of technology, birth itself has not changed. You, as a mother-to-be, still need to be prepared, nurtured and "mothered" by other women.

Instead of a baby shower, ask your friends to give you a Mother Blessing to celebrate your "birth" as a mother. The love and support in this kind of ceremony will boost your self-confidence.

All ceremonies symbolically destroy one world to create a new one. A Mother Blessing acknowledges the mother's new status, and also helps her say goodbye to the world she is leaving behind.

Around the world mothers are honored in many ways. In some

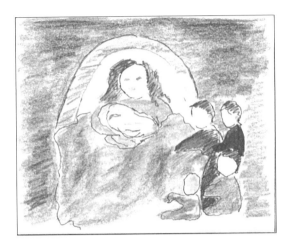

FIGURE 4.2 "I always birthed at night ... so the bed is half-moon shaped. The birthing woman is the centre of attraction, and the baby. She is covered with a pretty quilt. It's not really a quilt, but the beauty of birth. (The four figures in the lower right corner represent her husband and three children.)
Shannon

countries the mother, not the baby, is showered with gifts. My friend, Yoshiko, told me that in Japan there is a custom called Desire Day. On that day the pregnant woman can have anything her heart desires. Presents are again given to the mother thirty days after birth.

In Sudan, a woman is prepared for birth in her seventh month. Her hair is hennaed, braided and scented, and a special bracelet is worn on her wrist. She lies on a ceremonial wedding mat while friends gather around and rub handfuls of a vitamin-rich porridge on her belly to symbolize regeneration.[2]

Here in New Mexico, an expectant mum told me how she was "initiated" by a group of friends confessing "Bad Mum" stories. Everyone had to tell her biggest mistake as a mother. Afterwards they stood up and took a group "Bad Mothers" photograph. This unique and intuitive ceremony humourously eased the new mother towards feeling more connected, more human, and less anxious.

*

A STITCH IN TIME

My friend Sarah smiled all through her labour. She was amazing and radiant. At the end, when the pain became intense, she took a warm bath. I knelt by the tub and slowly poured water over her belly during contractions. In between contractions she told me the birth story of a pioneer woman she had read about in a quilting book. Thinking about that pioneer woman's courage in the face of unbelievable hardship strengthened Sarah's stamina and self-confidence. Not long after, Sarah gave birth to her first born, Laura, on the bedroom floor.

Later, Sarah gave me that book, *The Quilters: Women and Domestic Art*[5], and I read the story which had inspired her. It was told by Mrs. Wilman (in her 70s). While talking about her quilts she recounted the story her own mother, who settled on the high plains of Texas at the turn of the century, told her about making her baby quilt.

[My mother] used to tell me how when they come finally to homestead and the wagon stopped she felt so lonely. There was emptiness as far as the eye could see ... The houses was built underground and called dugouts. Or they would build a half dugout, finishing the top part with lumber and sod and tar paper ...

Muma's best quilts were her dugout quilts because that was when she really needed something pretty ... The butterfly [quilt] was free and fragile. It was the prettiest thing she could think of. She knew I was coming along and the Butterfly was for me ...

She didn't want a baby to be born in the dugout, but I was. And it was one more winter before they got above ground. She said she just wasn't gonna live underground with a baby, but they couldn't get crop or cattle money and the lumber was expensive.[5]

I was inspired by this story. During my second pregnancy, I made the Butterfly quilt for my baby. Stitch by stitch, quilting became a self-induction, connecting me with both the pioneer woman's gritty spirit and Sarah's smiling tranquility in her birth.

CREATING YOUR OWN MOTHER BLESSING

HOW TO BEGIN:

- Read about celebrations in other cultures and countries.
- Brainstorm with others. Make a list of everything you associate with celebrating a mother's rite of passage through birth. Blending your ideas will make for a richer event.
- Choose a theme, structure, and message.
- Pick out music that fits the ceremony.
- Look in cookbooks for recipes and cook up a special feast.[3]

A FEW MORE IDEAS:

- Form an intimate circle around the mother, making her the centre of attention and love throughout the ceremony. You could massage the mother, brush her hair and sing to her.
- Make a birth-blessing bracelet. Each woman brings a special bead to the ceremony. While sharing her blessing-wish with the mother, she strings the bead on the bracelet, and passes it on. After the ceremony, the mother wears the blessing-bracelet until labour is over, as a constant reminder of the blessings and support from her friends.
- As part of a ceremony, consider blindfolding the mother and taking her on a trust walk.
- You might include traditional raw materials for ceremonies: sage, cedar or sweetgrass for smudging, candles, incense, bubble or herbal baths, massage oil, face paint, or drums.
- Give the mother a fragrant, soothing herbal footbath. Float flower petals in the water. Gently dry and massage her feet.

- And for the more adventurous: organize a group belly dance. Belly dance originally was performed by women for a woman in labour to show her how to move the baby down and out.
- Reading inspiring stories, poetry, prayers, and blessings.
- Each friend takes a votive candle home from the Blessing and lights it as soon as she hears labour has started. The mother's awareness of those warm, flickering lights lit for her will be an added source of strength and comfort.
- Pass a yarn or ribbon around the circle, weaving it in front of and behind each woman, to symbolize the inter-connection and solidarity shared with the mother. Cut the string between each woman, and tie it around her wrist. This reminds each woman to think of the birthing woman and send her support in labour.[4]

MAKE A FRIENDSHIP CRIB QUILT: REVIVING THE QUILTING BEE

There's something about a quilt that says
people, friendship, community, family, home and love.

THE FOXFIRE BOOK

Although a friendship baby quilt can be a surprise gift, the hours spent quilting with women friends, laughing, gossiping, and sharing birth and mothering stories is a gift in itself? At a time when pregnant and working women often feel isolated, this warm event might be a highlight of your pregnancy.

Piecing and quilting your baby quilt will take at least a month, depending upon how many women are working it, and how quickly they quilt. The quilt should be finished a few weeks before your due date so your baby can be swaddled in it on its birth day.

HOW TO MAKE A BUTTERFLY QUILT

FINISHED SIZE IS 44 × 44 INCHES

- 1 yard muslin or solid cotton for nine squares, 11″ × 11″
- 1½ yards of contrasting fabric (print or solid) for borders
- 1¾ yards print fabric for backing
- Quilt batting and quilting thread
- Embroidery floss for antennae
- Bias tape: in several colours to border tops of butterfly wings; and 5 yards of one colour for border of quilt

WHAT TO DO:

If you haven't quilted before, consult a quilter or a book for instructions.

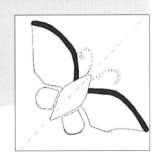

Because we are human,
Birthing from Within
is easier when we are enfolded
by the connection
and support of other women.

HERE'S HOW IT'S DONE:

The top of the quilt is made of separate squares and borders, or irregular pieces if it's a crazy quilt, sewn together. If squares are used, they should be identical in size; use any colour scheme that strikes your fancy.

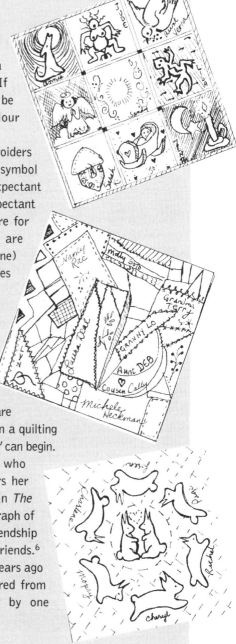

Each friend or relative embroiders or appliques (on a square) a symbol expressing her wish for the expectant mother, couple, or baby. The expectant mother can also make a square for the quilt. All of the squares are given to a friend (by the deadline) who has agreed to sew the pieces together to form the top.

Next, lay out the (ironed) material for the bottom of the quilt, wrong side up. Cover it with the cotton batting. Then, the pieced-together quilt, ironed flat, is laid evenly on top. The three layers are basted together and stretched on a quilting frame or ring. Now the "quilting" can begin.

Traditionally, each woman who helps with the quilt embroiders her name in the square she made. In *The Foxfire Book* there is a photograph of an elaborately embroidered friendship quilt, bearing the names of 55 friends.[6] It was made nearly a hundred years ago from scraps of material gathered from friends, and pieced together by one woman in a crazy quilt pattern.

Chapter 5

Eating in Awareness

> Even if you are the most calm, confident and determined
> woman in the universe, if you ignore proper prenatal
> nutrition, you're setting the stage for intrusive, possibly
> traumatic, birth interventions.

Peculiarly insistent, gnawing hunger pangs in the middle of the night are often the first sign we are with child. Right from the start, a thriving baby makes its presence known through its voracious appetite.

Throughout history, mothers have known (if not instinctually, then perhaps from folk wisdom) that eating well during pregnancy is a matter of life and death. Generations of mothers observed the connection between famines and miscarriages, stillbirths and other birth-related problems.

As part of humanity's collective unconscious, this knowledge shows itself in various cultural customs. In Poland, for example, it is a matter of common courtesy to offer a pregnant guest something to eat as soon as she arrives. When a pregnant woman in Greece expresses a desire for a certain food, people interpret this as a serious need of the baby and go to great lengths to obtain the item.

The medical world also has (conflicting) "customs" about prenatal nutrition. Imagine a continuum where at one end caregivers completely ignore the importance of what a mother eats, while at the other extreme, a particular, rigid, prenatal diet is made *essential*. A woman pointed in all these different directions may wind up being too dizzy to eat anything!

There is also disagreement about what is appropriate maternal weight gain. Some authorities prescribe a particular weight gain, often mindlessly restricting or increasing a mother's dietary intake to achieve that goal. Others emphasize proper nutrition rather than a specific weight gain.

Healthy pregnant women who neither restrict nor overindulge at mealtime can expect to gain 25 to 40 pounds, or even more, by the end of pregnancy. Weight gain patterns vary widely among pregnant women depending on their overall health, caloric intake, and metabolism. So don't worry about achieving a rigid month-to-month pattern of weight gain.

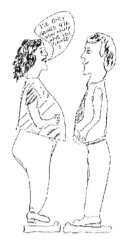

Joe portrays Being Pregnant *from a father's point of view.*

HOW CAN A MUM WITH AN ADEQUATE WEIGHT GAIN PRODUCE A LOW BIRTH WEIGHT BABY?

It's possible that a mother who eats a diet high in fats and carbohydrates, *but deficient in protein*, could gain a normal amount of weight, yet have a low birth weight baby. In this case, the mother's "adequate" weight gain is misleading; *she* is gaining weight on empty calories while her baby remains "hungry."

What's The Right Thing To Do? Keep your mind and your diet balanced and trust you'll grow a "just right" baby.

DINING WITH YOUR BABY

Eating is one of life's great pleasures, but some pregnant women lack an appetite or have concerns about gaining weight. If eating during pregnancy has become a chore (or your health care provider says that you need to be eating *more*), here's something fun that might help:

Every time you eat, make a mental picture of your hungry baby ... Imagine your baby munching along with you, bite for bite ... and that baby's kicking means "Yum, send down more."

"Hello, baby! I'm sending some juicy strawberries down ... I know you like these. Are you still hungry, you little thing? Do you want one more?"

BEING NATURAL IN MIND, HEART AND BODY

Listening to your body in the kitchen sets the stage for listening to your body in labour. Certain obstacles must be removed to permit such listening. The most common obstacle may be inexperience in being sensitive and responsive to your body's moment-to moment appetite.

It is nearly impossible to hear our stomach's inner voice over the din of fast foods, slick commercials, and trendy diets that drown out our intuitive knowing. Given this reality, sensitivity to our hunger and thirst must be consciously cultivated.

> "Food cravings are weird. It's like there's somebody in you ordering from their own menu. In my first trimester with Alex, I had to eat five bananas a day. Then one day, the order for bananas stopped coming."
>
> – RUTH

Good intentions do not always ensure a proper diet in pregnancy. Even when women want to eat properly, they may not know how. The majority of pregnant women I counsel *believe* they are eating well and are surprised to find out, through a diet assessment, that their daily protein, calorie, or vitamin intake is insufficient for pregnancy.

A woman may eat food which is healthy, but not enough of it. Or, she may over-emphasize certain food groups and neglect others (e.g., large quantities of fruit but insufficient "meat and potatoes").

TECHNOLOGY IS NOT A SUBSTITUTE FOR GOOD NUTRITION

If your health care provider does not provide nutritional counselling as part of your prenatal care, it may be that prenatal nutrition was not included in his/her medical education. Modern medical prenatal care emphasizes detection of problems in pregnancy, rather than their prevention.

These misplaced priorities are illustrated in the case of Becky, who was seven months pregnant when her doctor became concerned that her baby was not growing fast enough. He told her her baby was "at risk," and ordered a series of ultrasounds and lab tests, but did not ask her about her diet or low weight gain.

"Technology is not a substitute for good nutrition," cautions David Stewart in his book, *The Five Standards for Safe Childbearing*:

> No amount of prenatal blood sampling, urine testing, ultrasonography, amniocentesis, or other physical evaluations can substitute for good eating … All of these techniques and devices are for diagnostic information only. They do not heal. They do not treat. They do not assist the process of labour. They do not nourish. They do not prevent problems or complications.[1]

The notion of prenatal weight restriction is ingrained so deeply in our culture that Becky assumed it was the right thing to do. Without explicit nutritional counselling and encouragement to expect (and welcome) a weight gain between 25 and 40 pounds or more, a mother may deny her appetite in order to achieve the "right" results on the scales.

Becky was surprised to learn her pregnancy diet was severely deficient in protein and calories. With adequate protein and calories, Becky's baby feasted on the welcome abundance of nutrients now available. Two weeks later, her doctor was amazed at how the baby had grown!

As a result of this critical nutritional intervention, Becky and her baby continued to thrive. Two months later, she gave birth to a healthy seven pound girl.

> "It seems to me that the frequency of prenatal visits is opposite what it should be. Why aren't pregnant women seen once a week or every other week at the beginning of pregnancy—when counselling about diet and encouragement would make a difference in the health of the baby and preventing problems in pregnancy? Why check every week at the end, when it's too late to prevent or do much about problems that could have been avoided in the first place?"
>
> – EBONIE

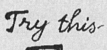

Try this

EATING THE
Universe

Whenever you eat·· when you drink
   milk·· be aware that
       everything in the universe
       is contained in the milk.

You will find sunshine, bees,
   clouds and rain
   that grew the grass
   the cow ate, the cow,
   and the farmer
   even dairy technology,
   in the milk.

Continue your meditation
   as you drink the
   "universal" milk.

Realize that this milk
   will become
   your blood and bones
   and the bones
   of your baby.

Practice eating mindfully
   with any meal.

If you're wondering whether you're eating too little or more than you need to, contrast your diet with the Common Sense Prenatal Diet at the end of this chapter. This diet is a guide, not a "should."

If you have a medical or special condition in pregnancy (see Appendix A), follow the diet prescribed by your doctor, midwife, or nutritionist.

PRACTISE EATING-IN-AWARENESS

Who you are in labour and as a mother is merely an extension of who you are in the rest of your life. So if you want to be present and strong in birth, you need to practise that way of being in your everyday life. The patterns of your life are all cut from the same cloth.

Eating is something you do every day, so practising eating-inawareness can prepare you for birthing-in-awareness. The way you are able to be *present* in ordinary day-to-day activities sets the stage for how you will be present while giving birth.

Thich Nhat Hanh is a Vietnamese Buddhist teacher and poet. A friend once asked him why he wasted his time growing lettuce when anyone could grow lettuce, but so few could write poetry the way he could. Thich Nhat Hanh's response to this compliment was, "If I do not grow lettuce [mindfully], I cannot write poems."[2] The following excerpt paraphrased from his book, *The Heart of Understanding*, expresses his way of living universal awareness in the moment:

If you are a poet,
you will see clearly that there is a cloud floating
in this sheet of paper.
Without a cloud there will be no rain;
without rain the trees cannot grow;
and without trees, we cannot make paper. So the cloud is in here.
Paper and cloud are so close …
the tree needs sunshine to be a tree.
If we look into this sheet of paper more deeply,
we can see the sunshine in it.
And if you look more deeply …

you see not only the cloud
and the sunshine in it,
but that everything is here;
the wheat that became the bread
for the logger to eat,
the logger's father—
everything is in this sheet of paper.[3]

You may be wondering how Thich Nhat Hanh's teaching is relevant to your prenatal diet. His view of life has helped some women realize the difference between eating mindfully and eating anxiously to meet daily nutritional requirements. As eating (mindfully) becomes part of your life, meeting your baby's nutritional needs will happen more naturally and pleasurably.

AN IDEA WHOSE TIME HAS PASSED (BUT NOBODY'S NOTICED)

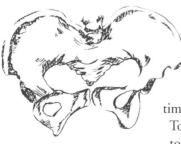

A normal pelvis.

A pelvis contracted by rickets.

The practice of restricting diet and weight gain during pregnancy got its foothold during the 19th century. It was introduced as a solution to an obstetric problem resulting from child labour practices of that era.

At the time, many European children grew up with poor diets and worked long hours in dark factories. The resulting deficiencies in Vitamin D and calcium caused a nutritional disorder called rickets, which impaired normal bone growth. A pelvis contracted by rickets often made birth more difficult, and sometimes life-threatening.

To help avoid tragedy in birth, doctors and midwives of that era recommended mothers eat less to try to grow a smaller baby, one that might more easily fit through a narrowed passage. Women who restricted their diet did produce smaller infants and increased their chances for surviving birth.

Rickets has become uncommon in the 20th century, and a severely contracted pelvis, for any reason, is rare. Nevertheless, the weight-restricting diet remained unquestioned as standard practice until recently. Researchers are finding that mothers with a poor diet and/or insufficient weight gain are more likely to have babies with a variety of problems. The mothers themselves face an increased chance of encountering several birth-related problems.

A GOOD DIET CAN HELP PREVENT:

- Anaemia
- Preterm birth
- Preeclampsia
- Foetal distress in labour
- Low birth weight
- Postpartum haemorrhage
- Mental retardation
- Learning disabilities

*

COMMON SENSE PRENATAL DIET

Rules can offer a sense of security. If rules help you feel comfortable, why not make some that will work to your advantage. For example, rather than create rules to restrict your diet, why not make rules restricting your rule making. Flexibility, not rigidity, characterizes a safe, healthy birth.

The Common Sense Diet is simply a guide, not a hard and fast rule to be followed.

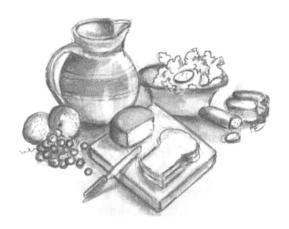

A COMMON SENSE DIET FOR PREGNANCY

DAIRY ... *4 choices/day*
    1 cup milk, yoghurt, sour cream,
    ¼ cup cottage cheese
    1 large slice cheese (1¼ oz.)
    1 cup ice cream

PROTEIN

MEAT ... *6–8 oz./day*
    Beef, lamb, pork, liver, chicken, turkey, fish, canned tuna or salmon

OR

VEGETARIAN ... *6–8 choices/day*
    Tofu 3 ½ oz
    Peanut butter/peanuts ¼ cup
    Beans ¼ cup + rice ½ cup after cooking
    Brewers yeast ¼ cup + rice ½ cup
    Rice ½ cup + milk ⅔ cup

OR

DAIRY AS PROTEIN—only consider milk as a protein choice if taken
in addition to your four milk-choices a day.
Cottage cheese ¼ cup
½ large potato + ¼ cup milk or cheese
Eggs
Tofu 3½ oz

FRESH DARK GREEN VEGGIES ... *at least once a day*
Broccoli, brussel sprouts, asparagus, salads, alfalfa sprouts,
spinach, etc.

WHOLE GRAINS ... *4–5 choices/day*
Slice of whole grain bread;
½ bagel; a pancake, waffle, or muffin
½ cup granola, any hot cereal or noodles.

VITAMIN C ... *one or two of these daily*
½ grapefruit or an orange
a large tomato or tomato juice
½ cup strawberries
green pepper

SALT TO TASTE

Salt sensors on your tongue have a higher threshold during pregnancy.
If food tastes flat it may be the salt sensors telling you that you need
more salt. So, unless you have heart or kidney problems, salting-to-
taste is another way of being in harmony with your pregnancy.

DRINK TO THIRST

Drinking about three litres of fluid a day helps your body to:
maintain the 50 percent increase in blood volume, and prevent
bladder infections, headaches and early contractions due to
dehydration.

The Art of Birthing

6

A Black Cloud Over Birth

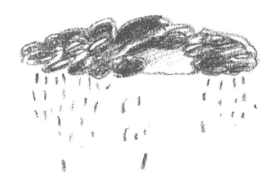

One of my early inspirations to write this book came from Annie, a young mother I met during my thesis research (studying the drawings of pregnant women in early and late pregnancy). Pregnant with her second child, Annie spoke favourably about her prenatal care, and was planning for a normal birth after Caesarean.

We began our second drawing session with this suggestion:

> Draw your image of *being* in birth. What is your image of what it will feel like to be *in* labour and birth? Your drawing can reflect an emotional, physical, imaginary or realistic experience. What is it like for you *being* in birth?

We were both shocked by the contrast between the image she drew and the positive feelings she had expressed only moments before. "I hope this labour is better than the last one," she said softly as she coloured in a blue patch along the lower border of the cloud. Leaning back in her chair to study her drawing, she slowly described how being-in-birth the first time was "like a black cloud" for her *(see above)*.

> I see a storm cloud. On the left it is really stormy, then there is a patch of blue sky in the storm … but it becomes stormy again. The left side of the cloud is the beginning of labour. It was very scary when I went to the hospital and they were doing so much to me. They started the IV, put on the monitor … and they broke my water right after I got there. Then they started the pitocin [syntocin drip] (to make the contractions stronger). I felt out of control, the doctor was in control. I was only dilated four and a half centimetres after all that. The blue patch is after seven to eight hours of labour when I was given Stadol and slept one hour … Suddenly, they came in and said I needed a Caesarean. It was stormy again.

Annie's image troubled me. I intuited the profound and larger meaning of her drawing and her loss. I felt uneasy as I sensed a question taking shape within myself: How could a woman whose image of birth was a threatening black storm cloud have the fortitude or self-confidence necessary for the kind of birth she was fantasizing?

While exploring her drawing, Annie tearfully disclosed how her disappointment and grief (over having a traumatic Caesarean birth two years earlier) had been discounted by her family and friends. They viewed the baby's health as the only measure of a good birth, and treated Annie's personal experience as irrelevant, if not trivial. Until our session, Annie had never brought up her feelings again.

Her drawing raised a second question: How were her childbirth teacher and doctor preparing her for this birth? She summarized what she was learning from the classes: labour physiology, the stages of labour, and various medical procedures the doctors might consider necessary during birth. One class was taught by an anaesthesiologist who explained a range of pain control options.

Like many women, Annie described her prenatal visits as an endless search for pathology. Even her baby, secluded in its sea of fluid, was not safe from extraordinary clinical scrutiny.

All this prenatal "care," but no one at the clinic or in her childbirth class asked her, not even once, about her hopes, her secret fears, or *her* vision of birth. Yet, insidiously her unresolved grief and self-doubts were affecting her body in ways which undermined her conscious plan to have a normal birth.

Since Annie was a research participant, there was no provision for therapeutic pursuit of the issues that had surfaced. *I* believe that, in the absence of therapy, the unresolved issues symbolized by Annie's "black cloud" contributed to her second Caesarean birth.

7

Birth Art Teaches

If you bring forth that which is within you, what you bring forth will save you. If you do not bring forth what is within you, what you do not bring forth will destroy you.

—GOSPEL OF ST. THOMAS

One kind of learning comes from books. But the learning necessary for you to participate completely in *your* birth must come from you. In making birth art or journaling, just bringing an image to light can be surprisingly revealing (and sometimes healing). Listening to it speak to you can tell you even more.

Dreams, reverie and art all carry messages from the unconscious. When exploring birth art, "We must," as Carl Jung observed in his discussion of imagery, "take the consequences of messages received."

An active, gentle exploration process not only brings overlooked resources and strengths to conscious awareness, but identifies obstacles and inhibitions that might prevent you from using them.

Birth art doesn't have to be pretty, colourful or carefully planned. It is as raw, honest, and spontaneous as birth itself. For example, when Renata was asked to draw *Being-in-Birth* (in her seventh month), she quickly sketched Figure 7.1. The drawing was the artistic equivalent of blurting out underlying anxiety.

What Renata was surprised to learn from her drawing was how angry she was that her doctor was not listening to her in prenatals, and how worried she was that he would not listen to her wishes in labour. She realized she was feeling trapped and helpless. After exploring this drawing, she made a decision to change her birth attendant.

*

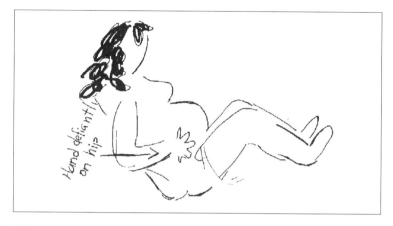

FIGURE 7.1 "Her legs are spread apart. She has red hair, and her hand is on her hip because she is angry. The words, 'Leave me alone,' refer to my recent burst of awareness that I could do it [give birth] if they would just leave me alone. I'm feeling defensive and annoyed about having to ward off intervention during labour."

It is important to notice how you approach making birth art because it is a metaphor for how you approach doing other things in your life, especially things you are unfamiliar with, such as birthing. Do you say, "I don't know how to do this" and hesitate, or give up altogether (leaving art-making to "artists")? Do you find yourself comparing and competing with the artwork of others? Or can you be curious and say, "Let's see what I can do?"

Your art, like your labour, doesn't have to be perfect. Just give it your best effort.

*

Most of us are used to communicating through language; usually that's the most effective form of communication. But through years of teaching holistic childbirth preparation I've learned that language has its limits.

A woman's birth story, myths or fantasies expressed in drawings can include details, affect, and symbols that might never be expressed in conversation. In drawings she is able to express vividly her inner-most beliefs, and recall perceptions and memories without confining them to the limitations of the spoken word.

Dream imagery, and the imagery expressed in art, both erupt from the unconscious and are explored in much the same way. Freud observed that "part of the difficulty in giving an account of dreams is due to our having to translate these images into words. 'I could draw it,' a dreamer often says to us, 'but I don't know how to say it.'"

We become conscious of any idea only after our mind's eye perceives the idea as an image. Although images are sketched through language, language can not duplicate the actual image. When described in words, an image is distorted because the three dimensional experience of an image can't be captured in a one dimensional form of communication.

In addition, we omit or minimize in communication those feelings or beliefs which our socialization has taught us are unacceptable.

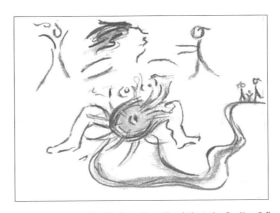

FIGURE 7.2 "After I saw what I drew, I realized that the [yellow] flames coming out of my uterus reflect an inner strength that will get me through the experience. The water-blue waves in my hair balance out the fiery strength with a tranquil security and confidence. On either side of me, I'm supported by Jorge and my own self: The birth experience will lead me into a new experience with my husband and new baby, who is illuminated by the power of life from the birth experience [in red, orange, and yellow pastels]."

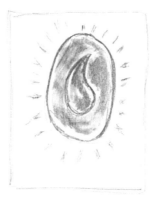

FIGURE 7.3 "The yellow rays around the womb are the life forces which the baby generates. I drew the baby as a drop of water, because it was the purest, most culture-less element I could think of. I tried to make the baby culture-less because I was thinking the other night how amazing it was that our baby thought of the world without the structures of language and culture with which we construct the world."

WHAT MOTHERS AND FATHERS LEARN FROM MAKING BIRTH ART

The response from parents who've made birth art is overwhelmingly positive. Over and over I hear mothers say that before making birth art, they had never thought about how they envisioned birth.

After class one night, first-time parents Hannah and Jorge expressed their gratitude for what they learned from their drawings. The mothers were asked to draw their *Strongest Image of Birth* while the fathers drew *A Womb With a View.* Hannah and Jorge admitted they were sceptical and uncomfortable entering into this exercise.

Hannah said, "Until I drew my picture (Figure 7.2) I could never envision giving birth. Every time I tried to read about what to expect in labour, I became anxious about what could go wrong and began crying. I'd turn my attention back to the chapters on pregnancy and taking care of myself. But when I finished my drawing tonight, I knew I could give birth. For the first time, I knew how to do it!"

Jorge had a difficult time making his drawing (Figure 7.3), but what he shared moved everyone in the class. "I am so close to this baby, it's hard to make a picture of everything I feel about it."

Jorge's reactions are not that unusual. Sometimes people who are left-brained, verbal, or thinking types initially are most apprehensive or uncomfortable about making birth art. Paradoxically, these people are the ones who often benefit the most.

Four things stand out from my work helping mothers explore their art. The first is that pregnant women unconsciously accept scientific and/or television images of birth. Few women acknowledge or even know what their own image of birth is. Yet it is *their* images, whether ignored or acknowledged, that will determine how they prepare for and experience pregnancy and birth.

Second, while exploring their birth art women often realize the value of spiritual and psychological support from other women during pregnancy and labour, and begin to seek or welcome that support.

Third, during the quiet, reflective process of making birth art, mothers become more aware of their unborn baby. They report more maternal feelings and a greater sense of bonding. And finally, women express gratitude to be heard, acknowledged and given time to reflect on their inner process.

*

As part of my thesis study of the drawings of pregnant women, I asked participants for feedback about their experience making birth art. A sample of their comments follows:

P.E.: Comment on your overall experience of the drawing session.
MOTHERS:
- "Incredible! … made me think of things I never thought of before. I got in touch with what was going on inside of me."
- "It was a process that helped me think more clearly about pregnancy, brought my pregnancy into focus."
- "It was fun … I was a little tense because of my performance anxiety."

P.E.: What was the most positive aspect of the drawing session?
MOTHERS:
- "Talking about the drawings, getting my feelings out."
- "I liked the idea of expressing myself in a way that allowed me to be totally free to do anything I wanted."

- "Made me think about what might happen."
- "The drawing sessions helped me work through some issues; it was a discovery process that helped me to solidify my intentions with this birth, helped me to visualize it."
- "I was anxious about labour and didn't know it. Using my head and hands got me in touch with it."

P.E.: What was most negative about the drawing sessions?
MOTHERS:
- "It was negative in a good way to realize I wasn't being honest with myself, I was going along with what was easiest for the clinic."
- "It was hard taking an image out of my mind, and putting it on paper."
- "Feeling uptight that it should look a certain way … wondering what other mothers drew."
- "I wanted brighter colours, especially water colours."
- "My lack of artistic ability."

P.E.: What did you learn from the drawings that was helpful?
MOTHERS:
- "Making drawings were helpful in connecting pregnancy to nature, it was very affirming. It was the only outside contact that validated me in pregnancy."
- "The sessions forced me to sit down so I could see my own images, which I would not have done without making the drawings."
- "Wasn't in touch with mothering feelings before I made the drawing."
- "The *Door To Birth* showed me women, not just my husband, could support me. I also became aware of my fear of looking primitive or needy."
- "It was helpful learning how to visualize labour."
- "Visualizing the birth helped me in birth. The head crowning picture came up when I was pushing."

8

Taking The Plunge

WHAT YOU WILL NEED: ART MATERIALS

You don't need to buy everything on the list to get started. Choose a few that appeal to you and begin.

- **PAPER:** Large paper encourages artistic freedom; try 11" × 17" or 18" × 24" drawing paper.
- **CRAYONS:** Get a box of regular size and try fat crayons, too—they help express the "big picture."
- **PASTELS:** A box of 8–12 colours. *NOTE:* These are a favourite. You may enjoy the soothing feeling of blending the soft, pretty colours with your fingers. You can also "paint" a pastel drawing with a wet brush.
- **PAINT:** Acrylic, watercolour, tempera or fingerpaint.
- **BRUSHES:** One or two big brushes will allow loose, free movement while painting (the same feeling and movement your body-mind needs in birth). Don't limit yourself by using those scrawny little brushes that come in the paint box!
- **COLOURED PENCILS:** There are soft and hard leads to choose from. Colours blend and shade more easily with soft leads. Some pencils turn to water colours when touched with a wet brush. These are great for journal work!
- **CLAY:** Basic grey clay is cheap and can be bought ready-to-use in five to twenty pound bags.
- **SCULPTING TOOLS:** You can buy an inexpensive set of tools, or use kitchen utensils (e.g., chopstick, garlic press, rolling pin, fork, spoon and so on).

WHAT YOU CAN DO

See how many ways you can creatively express and explore the following through Drawing, Painting, Sculpting, Writing, or even a Dance!

1. **PREGNANT WOMAN** How do you see yourself as Pregnant Woman?
2. **BEING PREGNANT** What is *being* pregnant like for you? (a physical experience, a spiritual feeling, a thought or even an abstract image.)
3. **FANTASY OF LABOUR AND BIRTH** What is your fantasy of labour and birth? (realistic or completely imaginary, physical or emotional)
4. **JOURNEY/LANDSCAPE OF BIRTH** Imagine your birth as a journey through a landscape; it could be water, earth, sky, forest, desert, or anything else. What's the weather like? What and whom would you want with you on your journey?
5. **DOOR TO BIRTH** If there were a secret door to birth, to giving birth, what would it look like? What's behind, around, or in front of it? Is anyone in the picture?
6. **THE OPENING** Create an image that will help your body relax, open, and bring your baby into this world.
7. **DRAWING ON YOUR ANIMAL NATURE** What animal do you associate with "easy birthing" or "good mothering."
8. **ARTIST-HISTORIAN** Imagine you are an artist-historian showing someone from another planet or culture what birth in our culture is like. Your assignment is to record in a drawing, or a series of drawings, how women give birth in this time and place.

   Draw the birth place and illustrate the customs. If there are people at births, show what they are doing there. Try to be objective. This may or may not represent your own birth expectations or values, but it should represent the current birth customs.
9. **DRAWING ON YOUR COPING SKILLS** Supposing you had done everything in your power to prevent or avoid a particular thing you fear in labour, and still it happened. Accept that you feel afraid. Then, imagine yourself coping with this

unwished-for event using internal and social resources. Draw yourself coping.

10. **A WOMB WITH A VIEW** Imagine you could take a peek through a window in your womb. What is your baby doing in his/her womb all day? What does he/she look like? See? Hear? Feel?

11. **CLOSING MANDALA** This project has been a big hit with parents during their last child birth class. Cut a circle, of whatever size seems best for you, out of cardboard, poster board, or foamboard. On it use collage, words, drawing, or painting to portray the following themes: the relationship between you and your pregnant belly, the unity between you and your baby, and/or the learning from class (or this book) you'll want to take with you.

TRY THIS:

BEGIN WITH A DOODLE

Doodling and scribbling are a good way to warm up your imagination and your drawing muscles. If you're not used to the art media, play with them and discover what they can do as you doodle. Following the instructions below, make a doodle using as many colours as you wish.

So, to begin, relax and let your eyes partially or even completely close. Become aware of the movement or stillness within you. What are you feeling in your body and heart at this moment? Is the sensation warm / cold, sluggish / alert, happy / sad, tense / soft or open / closed? Notice any thoughts that come up, then gently let them go.

When you are ready, take up your crayon, pastel or paint brush and begin flowing onto the paper. Let the movement or intensity in your body-mind match the movement as you work.

*

After you are finished, sit back and contemplate the doodle. What is the feeling in it? It may feel slow, fast, flowing or constricted.

Does this match what's happening within you? Just observe your doodle, don't critique it.

In one of his notebooks, Leonardo da Vinci wrote that one could find marvelous ideas by stopping to "look into the stains of walls, or ashes of a fire, or clouds, or mud or like places ..."[1]

Continue gazing at your doodle until you see an image (turn the paper around if necessary). Then outline or highlight it with a contrasting colour. Next, follow the gentle Exploration Guidelines in the chapter.

WHAT IF YOU CAN SEE IT, BUT CAN'T DRAW IT?

Ask yourself what you would draw, if you could draw very well. Describe that image. Taking up your crayon or paintbrush, where would you put the, say for example, tree ...?

Do it—Step by step, create the image.[2]

Even when your crude "masterpiece" is wildly discrepant from the polished image in your mind, the process of discovery, and perhaps healing, has unfolded. If you do get stuck while making art, it's a wonderful opportunity for learning. Some people think if they can't do something perfectly, they shouldn't do it at all. But in this exercise, as well as in your birth, it's your best effort that counts, not the attaining of some perfect image.

When asked to make birth art, some people feel intimidated by the difficulty of getting "from here to there." Imagining how you will get through labour can also seem intimidating. But remember—you don't have to get through a whole labour! You only can experience *one* contraction, *one* rest, *one* push —in any moment. Just as your labour unfolds one contraction at a time, allow your picture to unfold one stroke at a time.

Once a man who was 106 years old was asked, "What's it like to have lived 106 years?" He replied with a twinkle, "I don't know. I didn't live 106 years, I lived one moment at a time."

WHAT TO DO:

Before jumping into making birth art, take a few minutes to quiet your mind. Entering a meditative, receptive state, rather than a goal-oriented one, heightens creativity. Images which speak to us truthfully and eloquently surface when we are not trying to make them happen.

There is no need to bring anything extra to this process. Just as natural labour unfolds spontaneously, regardless of an individual's intention, so should making birth art. Bringing an intention to create something fantastic or original, or trying to impress some-one, does not enhance the process.

Although you can make and explore your birth art alone, it's best to work with a friend, counsellor, or a small group of women. Childbirth classes can be a natural group setting for practising these exercises and for involving fathers.

If you are working in a small group, initially refrain from talk-ing so that each person can go deeper into thoughts and imagery. If the desire to talk about something unrelated to your birth art arises, ask yourself if, and how, this distraction would be helpful. Maybe you are too close to an important feeling or memory, which you are reflexively avoiding. Making birth art mindfully can be the vehicle to that awareness. Afterwards, you can explore and talk about what came up.

Save your birth art. Date it and make a note describing the symbols, colours and what it means to you. Take any or all of your birth art to your birth room to inspire you. Later, you and your child might enjoy looking at what you made preparing for his/her birth.

A GENTLE EXPLORATION PROCESS

You have courageously pushed out
your image
onto paper or clay
Now Be Still
Let the image breathe and unfold
Before you name it.

- Stand back and quietly look at the art. Be curious. (If you wrote a poem or journal entry, read it aloud or listen to it be read to you.)
- Notice what you may not have seen at first.
- Concentrate on the feeling in the drawing or writing.
- What was the feeling when you were making this drawing / sculpture / poem / dance?
- Is there a story, a time, or place, behind this drawing?
- Is this the beginning, middle or end of the story?
- Was there anything surprising to you in this image?
- Is there anything that doesn't make sense to you?
- Is there anything you wish you had included in the drawing? What might that missing part mean (symbolize) about your life?
- Is there more? ... Draw or paint the next image in the story.

9

Discovery Through Drawing and Painting

In my research, therapy sessions, and classes, I often ask mothers (and sometimes fathers) to draw or paint one of the following six assignments to help them explore questions and prepare for their journey. You may appreciate seeing what other mums drew, and reading what they had to say about their images. But, to get the most out of this chapter—try doing them yourself.

I: PREGNANT WOMAN

> The relationship of mother and child is so simple
> that every peasant woman takes it for granted;
> so full of emotional content
> that artists, poets and story-tellers
> have been lured by it in every age …
>
> —M. ESTHER HARDING *THE WAY OF ALL WOMEN*

Using the *Pregnant Woman* drawing I explore pregnant women's self-image: how they perceive their physical and psychological being in pregnancy or as mothers. Here's what I ask them to do:

> Draw, paint or sculpt your image of *Pregnant Woman*. This image could be an abstraction or a human form, a self-portrait (or a drawing of their wife), or how you see pregnant women in general.

Parents' portrayal of *Pregnant Woman* creates a mirror in which their self-image and beliefs are reflected, allowing them to be seen clearly for the first time. This is beautifully illustrated by Nancy's work.

*

Nancy, a client of mine, was in the middle of her second pregnancy when she began exploring her beliefs, self-image and the possibilities for experiencing this birth differently. Later, she recalled how one session of making birth art had changed not only her self-image, but the course of her preparation for birth.

Her first birth, by Caesarean, had undermined Nancy's confidence in her body, and in trusting the natural process of birth. It was important to know how she saw herself now. To find out, we covered a huge cardboard refrigerator box with paper, and got out big brushes dipped in tempera paint. It was a warm day, so we worked outside.

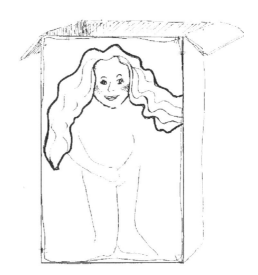

FIGURE 9.1

Nancy began by painting a figure with an elaborate face and flowing hair; the body was only sketched faintly (see Figure 9.1). Notice that the belly is small and guarded by her hands. (Hands guarding the pregnant belly is often seen when women have had a Caesarean birth, or fear one.) When she finished, she stepped back and reflected:

It's like looking in the mirror, because the paper is the same size as me. I am looking at how I see myself, at what I emphasize and make important. I can see I am more concerned about how things look, rather than how things are. I can see I am focused on how my body looks, appearances; I never realized I've been more concerned with having makeup on my eyes than what is going on in my belly.

With those insights, Nancy began painting over the original image, quietly exploring her emerging body- and birth-images (see Figure 9.2). When she finished, the new colours and detail emphasized her big belly, open vagina and her baby crowning. Her hands are lifted up, her legs are open and her face has a delightful expression of surprise.

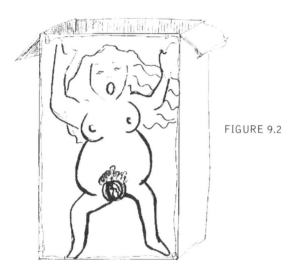

FIGURE 9.2

Looking at her paintings, Nancy commented excitedly, "Without these paintings I never would have seen this. I have *suddenly* shifted out of my head and into my body."

Nancy went on to give birth with her awareness in her *belly and pelvis,* instead of in her head. She gave birth to her son naturally, without inhibitions.

Years later, Nancy said of that realization, "That moment shocked me into reorganizing my priorities, which I continued to do over the next few months before I gave birth. That moment began a continuous process of drawing me out of my head and into my body, which I am still doing to this day."

*

Using the *Pregnant Woman* assignment, a woman can explore not only her pregnant body- or self-image, but also her physical and psychological adaptation to pregnancy. As women draw their image of Pregnant Woman, many comment on their first-time awareness of how they see themselves, or remember their own mothers.

Vanessa's flowing drawing (Figure 9.3) reminded her of "Rubens' women." Her feelings about the drawing and her pregnancy are "relaxed, comfortable and sensuous." Her drawing further conveys her experience of pregnancy as:

> … an overall voluptuous curve, … there's not enough paper … She needs to be big … Stomach should be bigger but then, I'm in my first trimester, and actually my breasts are bigger. I like the curves that happen when I'm lying down … would have liked to do my legs. She is faceless, because I am aware of my body changes, size, swelling.

FIGURE 9.3

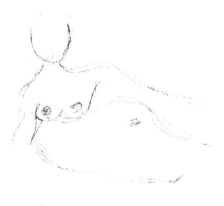

*

The next drawing is an example of a negative pregnant self-image (Figure 9.4). Before beginning the drawing session, Mary, a first-time mother in her first trimester, spoke positively about being pregnant. However, her drawing of a constricted pregnant woman, who did not even look pregnant, conveyed other feelings. Mary said:

> I used to think of pregnant women as cute and happy, but *I* don't feel cute. This is a self-portrait. It looks plain because before I got pregnant

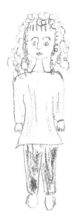

FIGURE 9.4

I had a figure. Still do, but clothes don't fit. I hate maternity clothes—
they're ugly. I drew a full head of hair to draw attention to her face
rather than her body.

Discovering such feelings might lead a mother to introspection, or
even therapy. But because Mary was a research participant, therapy
was not part of my working with her. For whatever reasons, Mary's
labour was long and difficult.

*

Self-image may be inferred from other kinds of drawings as well. For
example, a client of mine, Sarah, drew a row of colourful flowers
(Figure 9.5). Apparently she had been wanting to plant flowers that
spring, but thought she couldn't hoe the garden in her seventh month
of pregnancy. Exploring her birth art helped her realize that she'd
been seeing her pregnant-self as "weak and fragile."
    Symbols and images create their own reality in the body. A woman
who learns to view, and is viewed, as strong, capable, and protective

FIGURE 9.5

of her unborn, is more likely to birth well and begin motherhood with a positive attitude. Conversely, a woman who is induced to believe she is less than capable of growing and protecting her baby in pregnancy, or of withstanding the physical effort of labour, is more likely to depend on technology and others to reassure her, or to do it for her.

Challenging Sarah's "weak and fragile" self-image allowed her to discover untapped physical and psychological strength. This new view of herself gave her the energy to find a doctor who was more supportive of the kind of birth she wanted.

And she went on to plant her flower garden.

*

Paula, a warm and sensitive mother in my childbirth class, had had a previous traumatic labour resulting in an emergency Caesarean birth. When the class was asked to draw their image of *Pregnant Woman,* Paula drew a metaphorical "tree mother" in pastels (Figure 9.6).

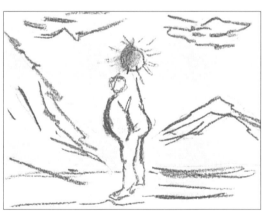

FIGURE 9.6

Here's what Paula told us:

> The green leaf is Pregnant Woman's body; the green represents growth. The brown tree trunk-legs symbolize strength. Her head is the sun; there is a bright feeling looking out to the horizon, to the unknown. The red in her body is her heart. There is no baby in the picture because we are all one. This is a happy pregnant person.
>
> The "tree" is how I felt about being pregnant the first time, before

the Caesarean. I wasn't afraid to give birth. I was *ready* to give birth. I *knew* I could do it. Don't get me wrong, I was scared of the unknown, of not knowing what labour would be like, but I knew I could do it.

After the Caesarean birth, she described herself as having been "very sad, just a sad feeling. Although I was happy to see my baby, I felt I never made a complete circle. Through circumstances, someone took it away, it never happened. I felt a loss, a guilt, sadness, a feeling I didn't make it."

However, Paula did not get stuck in the trauma of that birth experience and she reclaimed what she had always known to be true about herself and birth. "The tree image returned," Paula explained, "through therapy and the support of my husband."

After Paula gave birth to her second child normally, I asked her about her new self-image. She had this to say:

> This birth experience helped me find something I didn't know about myself. Going through the pain—and managing it, being in the trance … it was very powerful. For the next week I was still on a trip! I reviewed the birth over and over in my mind. Giving birth strengthened my essence of being. Through giving birth I found one more piece of who I am.

*

Like Stone Age artists, many women (even though unfamiliar with ancient Great Mother icons) draw *Pregnant Woman* or make sculptures that bear a striking similarity to the Stone Age icons! *Pregnant Woman* is portrayed as headless or faceless, with full rounded bellies and breasts, and thin or absent extremities.

Many women depict the pregnant body as just belly and breast (Figure 9.7)—and independently have similar reactions, commenting that a "pregnant body is headless because the head doesn't change when you're pregnant … can't tell if a woman is pregnant from the neck up. The focus is in her body."

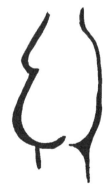

FIGURE 9.7

*

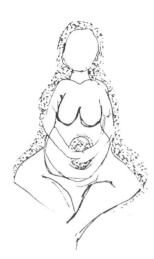

For some women, making birth art may be a reassuring affirmation of their readiness to give birth. Emma, an earthy 40-year-old artist, was about four months pregnant with her first child when she came to see me. When she finished her drawing of *Pregnant Woman* (see Figure 9.8), she spoke warmly about it:

FIGURE 9.8

Women are really wise. I feel the wisdom that's been waiting in me. There's faith that the body and woman are smart enough to figure out what to do. I was at my friend's birth a few days ago. I stood outside the room, listening. She made lots of different sounds. As I was listening, I realized that *women* figure this out. Their bodies figure it out. Of course, women have done this a long, long time.

This woman [in the drawing] is sitting in a relaxed posture. The blue halo [surrounding her body] represents her bond with other women around the world. Just as all of us, men and women, are touched by the air, we are all touched by birth. It's part of the link of humanity. Being pregnant has made me aware of it, of my link with humanity.

She is faceless because I was thinking of the commonality among all women becoming mothers that breaks all bonds; there is no hierarchy. And her head is brown to symbolize that the body is in charge. If I'm listening, I can hear the wisdom inside myself. I can trust my body.

*

Nikki, a mother in her fifth pregnancy, drew a particularly colourful and up-beat rendition of *Pregnant Woman*. She described her drawing in her warm, Texan lilt (Figure 9.9):

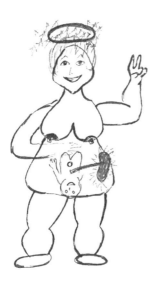

FIGURE 9.9

I made her muscled arms and legs for strength. My fingers are showing the "Victory" sign; overcoming self-doubts and difficulties in pregnancy and birth—you're victorious!

The purple halo and stars are for that airy-fairy feeling you get in pregnancy. I sometimes feel like I'm not connected to the world. We're angels when we're pregnant … not of this earth, yet at the same time I am 'cause pregnancy is so earthy. But the chemical changes in my brain make me feel off. My dreams and the things I think about, the way I think … are different [in pregnancy].

Every time I go in [for a prenatal] there's a question about what position my baby's in. So, I drew his head down to affirm he'll be in the right position. The placenta … this healthy thing is making my baby grow, it is part of me, part of my baby, yet separate.

2: BEING PREGNANT

Oh honey,
it's alright you cryin'
and don't know why.
Sometimes when a pregnant woman
is cryin' over nothin,
she cryin' for her baby 'cause it can't cry yet,
and when she laugh over nothin'
she laugh for her baby all happy in there.

—ADVICE FROM AN OLD AFRICAN-AMERICAN WOMAN

What *being* pregnant or a mother means to us is defined by cultural factors. The medical culture tells us that what's important about being pregnant are all the physical changes the mother and baby are going through. Mothers, wanting to do what's right, take the experts' cue about what's important. Not surprisingly, mothers begin to focus primarily on what they should *do* and *not do* to influence those physical changes (how they should eat and exercise, what they shouldn't drink, which tests they should take, and so on).

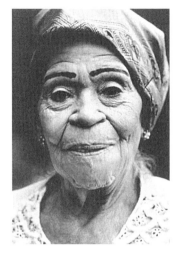

Photo credit: Lyn Jones

The birth-art used in advertising of baby products perpetuates the damaging myth that being pregnant and a mother *makes* a woman happy, calm, and fulfilled (which probably contributes to the soaring teen pregnancy rate). Those advertisements also define how we should feel and behave. When we predictably fall short of that unrealistic ideal, we feel guilty and inadequate. As a result, the ways we *are* coping successfully are devalued or ignored.

Contrasting sharply with the drug and formula companies' blissed out Polyanna-mother is *Smocked Figure* (Figure 9.10). Here, artist Judy Chicago captures the universal, natural experience of sadness and despair seldom depicted in birth art.

> While working on this image, Mary Ewanowski was reminded of a story her mother told her. Mary was the third of five children born to a Catholic home. Her mother tried to uphold the doctrine of the Church. "One day she told me that when she found out she was pregnant for the fifth time, she cried."[1]

In *The Women's Room,* Marilyn French describes pregnancy as "a long waiting in which you learn what it means to lose control over your life."[2] I wondered what pregnant mothers would say if asked what *being* pregnant was like for them. I gave them these instructions:

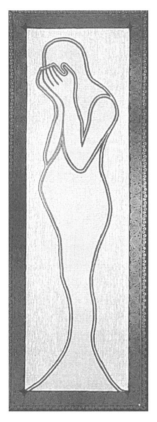

Draw a picture that expresses what *being* pregnant is like for you. This could depict physical experience, a spiritual feeling, a thought or even an abstract image. Sometimes your picture can tell a whole story, or just a moment, in the story of being pregnant.

The most common symbolic themes were change, obstacles, identifying with nature, personal strengths, and spirituality.

For example, Figure 9.11 is a crayon drawing made by a mother in her second pregnancy. She portrayed *Being Pregnant* using a series of images spanning from her previous Caesarean birth to a future image of "relief" postpartum. Her images include symbols for both obstacles and resources, and in her discussion of the image, she conveys her underlying anxiety related to integrating work, home, and becoming a mother again:

FIGURE 9.10 © Judy Chicago, 1984 Needlework by Mary Ewanowski, Chico, CA.

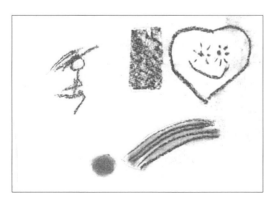

FIGURE 9.11

I feel anxious … running to get to the end of pregnancy [represented by the red wall] I have to stop and realize "It's a wall." It's not the unknown, it's not all fun and games. Stop and Prepare!

In spite of the past, my problems and present anxiety, the reality is [represented by the heart] I still feel content. I feel happy, full of love, looking forward to it.

There is light at the end of the tunnel [yellow circle]. The light represents that it's not as bad as it seems, not as tough as Christmas shopping, day care problems, work. Because of the pregnancy, I see light, see change coming. Pregnancy is like the light.

The rainbow symbolizes finding the pot of gold … which symbolizes the calm after the storm. [This is in reference to her boss whom she felt had reduced her responsibilities at work because he viewed pregnancy as fragile].

Figure 9.12 is a watercolour by Lilly, a mother in her third pregnancy. She had two previous healthy pregnancies and home births, and felt genuinely positive about mothering.

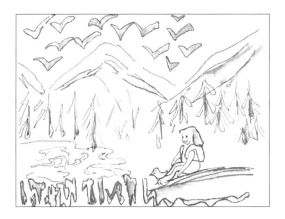

FIGURE 9.12

I feel like I want to put the whole world on [the paper]. Is that okay? My feeling is that *this* is God. The world created where people have not harmed it. The world is continuing through pregnancy. There is natural order, right, correct … in tune. I am happy, not sick, not down … Pregnancy is really important. This is at Nambe Lake.

The birds in the sky represent freedom, and the bird sitting next to me is an ally, a friend visiting. There's a smile on its beak. The sunny sky-radiance, illumination; the mountains represent earth, solid, stable, actually moveable in time; the rocks are the bones of Mother Earth, the spine of the earth sticking up into the air. The evergreen trees are Earth's hair.

3: FANTASY OF LABOUR AND BIRTH

In the first trimester, most women aren't thinking about labour or giving birth. Nonetheless, I've learned that it's worthwhile to ask them what their fantasy of labour and birth is. There are no right or wrong fantasies; whatever the mother draws enables both the mother and me to see the beginning point from where we'll launch our birth preparation work together.

In my study of the drawings of pregnant women, 14 of the 16 women who drew this assignment were planning to birth in the hospital, but only two included hospital symbols in their fantasy of birth. Many women reported blocking out the distractions they anticipated in the hospital so that they could focus on their birth and birth companions. Sometimes mothers will draw the baby and family *after* the birth. Part of birth preparation work is recognizing which material shouldn't be pushed out of awareness (see Chapter 20, "Even Paper Tigers Can Bite").

Everyone has a dream, a fantasy, even a fear, about what their birth will be like. Here's what I invite mothers to do:

> Make a drawing that depicts your fantasy of labour and birth. It can be realistic or completely imaginary; it may express the physical, spiritual or emotional aspects of birth.

Christina, a first-time mother who drew Figure 9.13, was very excited about becoming a mother. In her *Fantasy of Birth* she envisioned being in the hospital, represented by the symbol of a rigid, stark table/bed, yet her *focus* is on spiritual support:

> I picture myself in a hospital bed, in a wonderful position. There are lots of hands on me helping me get the baby out … cheered on by God [upper left, the hands and face—in purple] …The hands are real

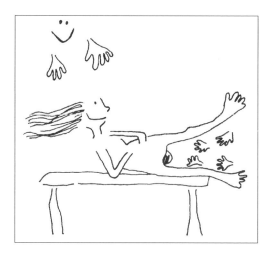

FIGURE 9.13

ones, and spiritual ones, maybe even my own … maybe that's why I didn't put them on me. I picture the room with subdued lighting, purple light, God smiling down on me. I'm aware of just my body, excited and awed.

4: BEING-IN-BIRTH

One of the psychological tasks of the third trimester is to prepare for the actual birth. At this time women's attention is turned toward learning about the physiological process, medical management and "breathing techniques."

Mothers learn from health professionals and childbirth educators what being *at* a birth looks like (or what professionals *do* for you in labour and birth). That's the perspective a health professional knows best—and that's what they teach.

But mothers aren't *at* their births, they're *in* their births: they're *in* labour, *in* a trance, *in* their body, *in* pain, *in* joy!

I wanted to help women explore their images of giving birth from that inner perspective. Here are the instructions:

When you think about being in labour, what image comes to mind? How does it feel for you to be giving birth? This drawing could express an emotional, physical, imaginary or realistic experience.

Being-in-Birth drawings are often abstract. Who can express *being* in the mystery of birth? Shelly, a spunky, determined participant in the study, made a bright, colourful abstract pastel drawing (Figure 9.14).

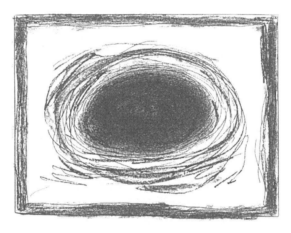

FIGURE 9.14

In our session, Shelly tearfully recalled being unsupported and lonely during her first hospital birth. In planning a home birth this time, she makes reference to "an environment that will support me this time." Her commentary captures the elusive, immense experience of birth:

Being in birth is beauty, bright, and bold ... soft and powerful. The uterus is the focus, all the energy goes there. Red is for intensity, in the center.

More pastel shades on the outside represent being relaxed on the outside.

Purple is for the strength of birth, the strength of the mother, the strength of the birth which is out of her control yet controlled by her strength.

Green is anticipation ... Something will come of all this intensity. The purple frame is the strength of the environment that is going to support me this time, and not detract from my birth.

5: JOURNEY/LANDSCAPE OF BIRTH

> Imagine your birth as a landscape; it could be water, earth, sky, a forest, desert, or something else. What's the weather like? What and whom would you want with you on your journey through the landscape of labour?

This assignment is a powerful tool in helping women transcend the limited (and limiting) image of birth as merely a medical or physiological event. The use of metaphor invites women to think of labour and birth in a fresh and new way, which creates an opportunity for personal awareness.

Following are three examples of landscape-journeys. The first drawing was done in crayon by a mother late in her second pregnancy (Figure 9.15).

When you look at the picture, what is the feeling-tone you sense within it? What emotions do you feel within yourself? The artist-mother slowly and quietly described her image:

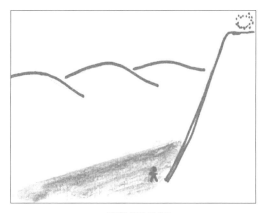

FIGURE 9.15

Labour is difficult and imposing. The sun [upper right on top of the mountain] is the light at the end of the tunnel. The hills represent the ups and downs in pregnancy. The pregnant woman is me—looking at what's coming. The shadow of the mountain coming over you … it's coming, the dread.

I dread the not knowing, not knowing the length of labour, the problems, the pain. The journey is straight up, the shortest way. Only one way to go, have to go. There's only one way to go to have a baby. I can control breathing, but I can't control anything else.

I'm alone. In the end you're alone. The Lord can help you but can't come down and do it for you. You're the one who gained the weight, gets stitches, can't sit …

I was thinking, wondering about where the birth was in the picture … It's where the light is [upper left]. After the birth, the mountain goes uphill a while [can't see the mountain ascend because she ran out of paper].

Then you journey down the other side of the mountain. When you get home, there's more mountains, up and down— that's how life is.

Drawings like this alert me to the possibility of prenatal and postpartum depression. The childbirth preparation of such mothers includes accessing and developing personal, family, and social resources. Without the information which surfaced in the drawing, this vital preparation might have been overlooked.

*

In the second example (Figure 9.16), you will notice a much different mindset than in the preceding example. Although this mother had never had a baby, her vision spanned through pregnancy, labour, and the first few weeks postpartum.

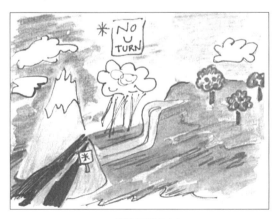

FIGURE 9.16

Early pregnancy is on the road where it enters the picture [lower left], the road brings you closer to labour. I like mountains. Climbing mountains is a lot of effort. There is a sign, a "No U-Turn" sign, because there is one choice, one way to the other side of the mountain. The rain and muddy place is when it's not real pretty for a while. It's where the birth takes place, in the middle of the road.

The dusty field is for hardship, need to pass through to get to good times ahead. I anticipate the first few weeks to be hard, then it will get better.

I like the colour purple, I associate bright purple with moods. This shade of purple is demanding it get noticed.

The fruited plains (laughter) … the fruit is non-specific, not aware of a special association. The snow I associate with cold and hardship. We used to live in the snow. There is danger and effort … but I don't suspect any danger or problems with this birth.

*

In the last example (Figure 9.17), Amy envisioned her impending labour as "a passage, a journey … the water is not calm, but not too rough. The boat represents me in labour, just going along, not interested in expressing, just feeling."

Amy added insightfully, "the blank space is all that we don't know."

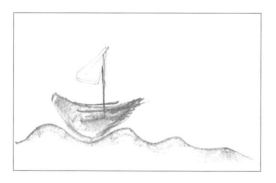

FIGURE 9.17

6: DOOR TO BIRTH

This drawing assignment is a favourite of most women. Like the Landscape/Journey assignment, the *Door To Birth* also taps the power and creative ambiguity of metaphor. The instructions are:

> If there were a secret door to birth, to giving birth, what would it look like? What's behind it, around it, or in front of it? Is anyone in the picture?

The "New Mexico Birth Door" (Figure 9.18) is a candid image drawn by a first-time mother who recently had moved to New Mexico, and was taken by the western ambience. She described her drawing:

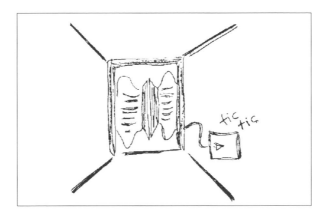

FIGURE 9.18

There's a timer to control the hinges [lower right] … When the force [of labour] and the mother and baby are ready … the door will swing open. This force is like a locomotive …

[She had recently attended a friend's home birth and was awed by it, observing that] the woman didn't have a whole lot to do with it. There was this force she had to work with. When she got to the "door," it swung open.

A woman can find a way around the door, that's why it's open above and below, she can have a Caesarean, go under it instead of through it … but the door can't be opened until the force arrives at it.

I wondered if her comment about going "under the door instead of through it" reflects the misguided notion that mothers who have Caesarean births have, or choose, the "easy way out."

Although this mother had a very long, difficult labour, she did not become discouraged and accepted the difficulty rather matter-of-factly.

Here are two more examples of *Door To Birth.*

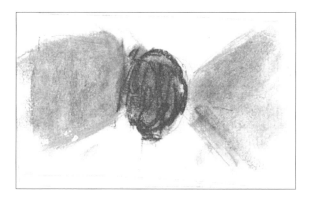

"It's a big door with flesh tones on both sides. The baby's head is behind the door — it opens the door. I'm in front of and behind the door. I have to help and allow the baby to move through it."

—TINA

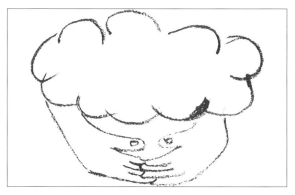

"My image is of two huge hands coming down from heaven, from heavenly clouds. The hands are helping, they are God's hands ... working just through faith. A lot of prayer will help the process of labour, and help the doctor make the right decision. "His" hands might be holding the doctor up ... it might be 3 a. m.. I should put the baby inside the hands—to show the process of birth.

—SHAWNA

10

How Birth Art Helped Donna Become A Mother

We can only speculate about the impact of positive self image on birth outcome. With a little encouragement and care, more mothers might begin motherhood with a positive attitude. This is illustrated in Donna's story, which unfolds in a series of drawings made throughout her pregnancy.

Pregnant for the first time, Donna simultaneously experienced excitement about having a baby and doubt that she would be a good mother. Her feelings of inadequacy surfaced in several of her early drawings.

In our first session, I asked Donna to draw her fantasy of birth. She drew a picture (Figure 10.1) of her new family *after* the birth, "In the country … because the birth itself is hard to imagine."

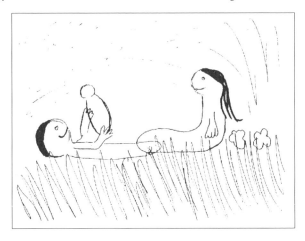

FIGURE 10.1

It is not uncommon for first-time mothers who have never seen birth to have some difficulty creating a clear fantasy image of themselves giving birth. However, it is noteworthy that Donna's mother figure, representing herself as a mother, lacks certain feminine or maternal attributes, and that the father is holding the baby.

While exploring this drawing, she remembered that her father abandoned the family when she was two years old, and her mother did not have the energy or resources to nurture her. These events shaped Donna's inner map of mothering and family life. Donna suggested that the father holding the baby in her drawing conveyed her hope that her husband would have a close relationship with their child, along with her doubts that she would be a good mother.

*

In another drawing (Figure 10.2), Donna is holding the baby at arm's length, and again portrays herself without hair, breasts or maternal attributes. This might suggest Donna was still arm's length from bonding with her baby. In the time remaining before her birth, she continued to explore and discover her inner resources and strengths as a mother. Focusing on becoming a mother in this case was far more important than "birth preparation." A woman who does not see herself as a mother, no matter how much she knows about birth, may have additional trouble surrendering to the hard work of labour.

Donna's growing confidence is shown in a later drawing (Figure 10.3). Note the maternal, feminine features in this self-portrait, and that she is nursing her closely-held infant.

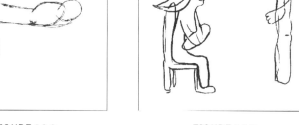

FIGURE 10.2   FIGURE 10.3

*

But there was still the problem of not having a mental picture of herself giving birth. I asked Donna to make another drawing of her fantasy of birth, but to move a little closer to her image of giving birth. She used a pale blue crayon to make Figure 10.4. The straight lines represent her thighs, the figure "8" is the baby. This is her story about the drawing:

> I just had the baby. The drawing is from my perspective, looking down I see my baby … The purple rainbow is my seeing. I feel happiness, fear, surprise and amazement.

*

I wondered how Donna envisioned the natural process of labour. I asked her to make a picture showing how labour worked (Figure 10.5). She drew a closed cervix first [upper left]. As she looked down on the paper, she talked sadly about her fear that she wouldn't be able to open.

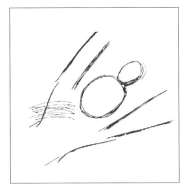

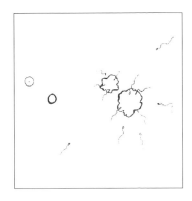

FIGURE 10.4   FIGURE 10.5

"Suppose you have been labouring for a while, and made some progress. What would your cervix look like?," I asked. She drew a thick rigid cervix that was "dilating to about 2 or 3 centimetres." (Don't these cervixes look like textbook illustrations?)

"Suppose a miracle happened, and you could open easily, all the way. What would that look like? What would it take to make that happen?"

Donna drew the dilating cervix [in a series of two on the right] in fuchsia pastel. The sperm-like shapes are hormones working on the cervix to help it change.

Donna was very pleased and visibly more relaxed after making this drawing.

*

As Donna's mother self-image became increasingly healthy and positive, she gained the confidence to make choices related to her prenatal care and birth. She had been dissatisfied with the prenatal care she was receiving, but needed to explore her own beliefs and strengths before she could choose an alternative birthing option that better matched her needs.

Here's what she had to say about her drawing, the *Door To Birth* (Figure 10.6):

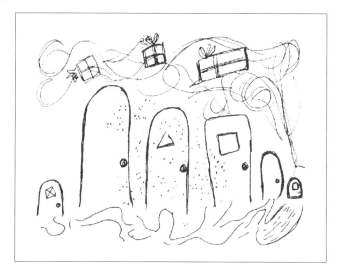

FIGURE 10.6

There are a lot of different paths leading to various doors representing birth options. Planning my birth is like going through a maze, having to pass by many big and inviting doors. I found the one secret door. The door is small because so few women choose it, it's so hard to find, and there are so many barriers. It's harder to create a normal birth experience [at home] because it's against the system's way of doing it.

It's a struggle to do what you want. It was hard for me to find my way. The gifts are presents from women I've been close to, gifts like strength to find what I wanted and the notion of women working with each other in birth.

*

In our final session, shortly before she gave birth, Donna's drawing of herself as "Birth Mother" undeniably mirrored her new self-image as a confident, capable and powerful mother (Figure 10.7).

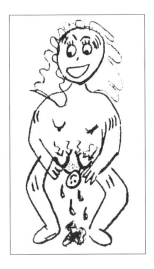

FIGURE 10.7

When comparing this drawing with earlier drawings, several important differences stand out. Out of approximately 20 drawings, "Birth Mother" is the first one in which she is facing forward, rather than a side view, and it is the first time she is standing, rather than sitting or lying down. This may represent Donna's experience of *being* more active in her birth process, or of her having *taken a stand* on how she wanted to give birth.

In all of her earlier drawings, there is a mild to gross distortion of the body, i.e., missing limbs, no hair or facial expression. In "Birth Mother," not only is her body whole, but she includes marvelous details, such as eyelashes, fingers, breasts, an open vagina and a look of surprise on her face and a smile on the baby's! She embraces the natural movement of birth illustrated by black motion lines on the face, arms and legs. The wavy fuchsia arrows pointing downward on her abdomen indicate the baby's way out. She even includes normal bleeding.

Donna gave birth normally to a healthy baby girl, whom she loves dearly.

*

Exploring your self-image is a journey which can bring you to a wonderful place, but may involve sweating, pushing and crying along the way.

ANCIENT SCULPTURES

Prehistoric peoples' awe at the mystery of pregnancy and birth is reflected in the exquisite form and power found in their birth art. One of the most beautiful images, the Goddess of Luassel (c. 19,000 B.C.), is carved on a limestone slab at the entrance to a rock shelter in Dordogne, France. She holds in her raised right hand a bison horn with 13 notches etched into it. The notches may represent lunar months. Her left hand points to her vulva or rests on her swollen, pregnant belly. Traces of sacred red ochre, the colour of menstruation and birth, are still visible on her body.

Of the hundreds of Stone Age sculptures known to us, only five are male figures. The predominance and wide distribution of the Great Stone Age Mother throughout Eurasia during the first 200,000 years of human history is dramatic evidence of her significance in human development.

The most common images of the Goddess were headless, sightless, or with her head inclined toward the middle of the body. The icons are typically rounded vessels, with a gigantic belly and breasts. Her arms are only suggested, huge thighs taper to thin legs, with no feet, or feet that were too fragile and small to have survived intact.[2]

The Great Mothers still exude a quiet power and exemplify the ancient perception of pregnant women as big and strong.

Anthropologists Sjoo and Mor remind us that 2–3 million years of human survival can be attributed to women's physical strength, noting that "the human race couldn't have survived ... if women had been as physically weak and mentally dependent during those hard ages as we are supposed to be today."

11

Revelations Through Clay

I like picturing connections in my head.
I am making my connection with clay.
Clay turns me on and it turns me in.
It seems clearer and clearer
that I was drawn to clay
by its plasticity.
For it is plasticity I seek in my life.
To be able to move into new and deeper forms …
in which I make the connection between
the life I'm living and the objects I'm forming.

—PAULUS BERENSOHN *FINDING ONE'S WAY WITH CLAY*

It was during my thesis research that I excitedly discovered a potential connection between mothers across millennia: expressing birth images through art! Initially I had formed an inaccurate image of ancient Great Mother figures as hefty, impersonal statues chiseled out of boulders. Then one day I saw a replica of the Goddess of Willendorf in a museum. It was small enough to be held in the palm of a hand! From that moment I viewed the pregnant goddess figurines as *intimate*, personal fetishes.

While we can only speculate about what meaning and purpose they had for *ancient* women, I instantly envisioned the possibility of *modern* mothers making personal birth-power sculptures as part of their childbirth preparation. This simple, creative activity not only helps pregnant women realize their connection to an unbroken chain of mothers, but also helps women see, feel, and speak their innermost beliefs.

Sinking their fingers into moist, malleable earth seems to take women to a deeper, unconscious, earthy kind of knowing. As they pensively shape a meaningful symbol out of a lump of clay, they often bring to light inner wisdom or unrecognized beliefs about birth and motherhood.

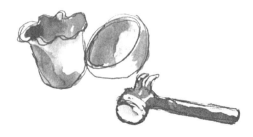

Betsy made a hammer. "It just made itself." She couldn't say what it meant, as she looked around and saw all the mother figurines and rattles. "But my clay would not be a rattle, it wanted to be a hammer!" She thought about the hammer symbol all week and reported it meant she "was building something here, a baby, a family, a new life."

Holding their "truth" in hand, mothers (and fathers) more readily share with others their new discoveries about themselves. Thus a too often passive learning process in childbirth classes becomes an active, creative effort, shifting from a teacher-knowing to a *mother*-knowing group.

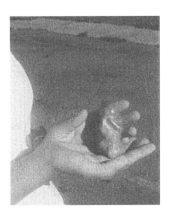

This sculpture, made by a father, was originally a baby in a womb or a crib. After class, he continued to work on his sculpture. Before they had a chance to fire it, his wife went into labour. She rubbed the baby-sculpture with her thumb through thirty hours of labour, rounding the edges and burnishing it to a shine. Later, showing it to me in my office, she handled it with the care usually shown a Ming vase.

This exercise quickly became a favourite in my childbirth preparation groups. Although traditional childbirth classes don't include this kind of exercise, mothers and fathers can make birth sculpture on their own or with friends.

FATHERS' SCULPTURES

When I first introduced making birth art in childbirth classes, I assumed fathers would not want to participate. I was wrong; fathers often plunge right in.

I explain about birth-power sculptures to the group and give each a lump of clay. Then, I send the mothers to work in one room, while the fathers and birth companions stay with me to explore reactions and roles in the birth process. Upon reuniting, everyone talks (with great animation!) about their sculptures.

I've been surprised by the connections or similarities couples' sculptures sometimes have. For example, several times mothers have made a swaddled baby and were delighted to discover that their partner made a cradle (that fits!). Sometimes both partners have sculpted nearly identical shapes or symbols. Fathers often bring their wives the gift of humor by making clay "brass" knuckles to "fight the pain," or "be tougher than the pain," or a screwdriver to remind her "to open up in labour."

THE POWER OF BIRTH SCULPTURES IN LABOUR

The vivid realizations that come from making birth art can influence future behaviour much the way hypnotic trance is used in therapy. The emotional depth of "knowing" arrived at through making, exploring and using personal birth art brings with it the potential to influence behaviour in the moment. I have watched women in labour hold, squeeze, rub or gaze at their birth sculptures, recalling the empowering awareness they had while making them.

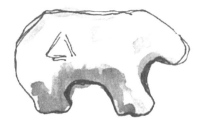

Bears are a symbol of good mothering. Native Americans make bear fetishes for healing.

BIRTH-POWER SCULPTURES BECOME HEIRLOOMS

When your child is grown you can pass down the birth-power sculpture that helped you bring him/her into the world. Not only is this another thread connecting the generations, but it also begins the process of your child's preparation for his or her rite of passage into parenthood.

WHAT YOU WILL NEED:

1. Grey or Red Clay—is cheap and can be found at ceramic supply and art stores.
2. A Clay Tool Set or Kitchen Utensils—to help shape or decorate sculptures, e.g., rolling pin, chipstick, ice pick, fork, knives, garlic press, and small sponge to smooth the surface or moisten the clay.

WHAT TO DO:

It is most beneficial to you to approach this activity as another practise in mindfulness rather than an art making project. Throughout this process, practise "listening" to your unfolding process, moment-by-moment, without directing it.

Begin quietly holding the lump of clay in your hands, *feel* it resting in your hands. Notice your breathing. Notice how ideas about the sculpture or the upcoming birth come and go in the mind. Bring your attention back to your breath and notice ideas move in and out of the mind.

When your mind becomes quiet, begin working the clay until all the air bubbles are out and the clay is malleable. As you knead the clay continue to pay close attention to your outward breath. Feel the clay: if it seems a bit dry, dip your fingers into a small bowl of water or vinegar to moisten it.

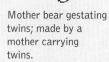

Working the clay into your hands, notice how forms naturally emerge and sink back into the lump (just as thoughts and images come and go in the mind). When a shape or symbol emerges that captures your attention, work the clay to bring that image out. It won't necessarily make sense to you or be what you "had in mind."

Mother bear gestating twins; made by a mother carrying twins.

Sometimes it happens that while working the clay, a clear image or symbol will surface in the mind—intentionally sculpt it into the clay.

After the sculpture feels complete, contemplate what has taken shape. What emotion or feeling was evoked as you made it, and what is arising as you look at it now? If the sculpture could talk, what would it say to you? Did it surprise you?

If you decide to save your sculpture, set it aside to dry for a week to two. Sculptures at this stage are called *greenware*, and are a bit fragile. To make sculptures resistant to breakage, fire them in a kiln. If you don't have one, ceramic stores will fire for you for a minimal charge. Grey clay fires into a beautiful bone white. If you want colour, you can paint with an underglaze before firing, or paint with acrylics *after* firing.

HOW TO MAKE YOUR BIRTH SCULPTURE

SCULPTING IN-THE-MOMENT

Childbirth is unpredictable. We try to gain "control" by planning and making decisions ahead of time. We tightly hold onto whatever makes us feel safe or confident. The ideas that don't fit into an "acceptable" frame of reference may be actively denied, or, more subtly, allowed to drift out of awareness.

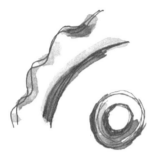

Brass knuckles to "fight fear or pain."

The ring to symbolize cervical dilation.

While all of your planning may spin a cocoon of security, in actuality the course of your labour is unknowable. As a mother-to-be, your critical task is to prepare for a birth that has *no* script. This requires great courage, flexibility, and a capacity for inner awareness. You can begin *now* by practising being open and responsive to each moment in your life as it unfolds. Paradoxically, one way to learn this is to notice how you are *not* being open and responsive in the moment.

Another way to practise being in the moment is making a series of birth sculptures from the same piece of clay. Begin by working the clay and emptying the mind. Then sculpt for five minutes. Take a look at the sculpture; contemplate the symbol and its meaning for you.

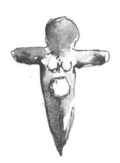

Carol's sculpture "shows a symbol of [her] faith, the mother is laid out like Jesus on a cross. But this is a mother, it is Eve and Mary, she has a belly which is my baby. I will think of those women when I give birth."

A sculpture, no matter how extraordinary it is, captures the awareness or insight of the moment. It is inevitable that perception, understanding and symbols change over time. So view each of your sculptures as a catalyst, *at that moment*, to help you investigate ideas that are influencing or restricting your birth as a mother.

When ready, fold the sculpture back into a lump. Repeat the process several times.

During this birth art exercise, pay close attention to your reaction (or resistance) to smashing your sculptures. Be aware of what happens when your mind latches on to a particular sculpture or the meaning you've given it; notice when there is a reluctance to let go of a sculpture. How is your response different when you're obliterating a sculpture you didn't like?

I suggest there is a correlation between your response to creating, smashing or saving sculptures and what happens with ideas (you create) about pregnancy and birth. Throughout the exercise, practise equanimity with the sculptures and your ideas: soften around all your ideas and judgements.

> … because I know I am made from this earth,
> as my mother's hands were made from this earth,
> as her dreams came from this earth
> and all that I know, I know in this earth,
> the body of the bird,
> this pen, this paper, these hands,
> this tongue speaking,
> all that I know speaks to me through this earth
> and I long to tell you, you who are the earth too,
> and listen as we speak to each other of what we know;
> the light is in us.
>
> —SUSAN GRIFFIN *WOMAN AND NATURE*

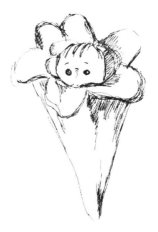

"I want a reminder to open up like a flower ... instead of ripping and tearing. I'm gonna open like a rosebud. That's my baby being born."

—MARY

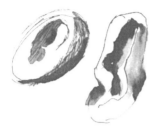

Many women make ''rubbing stones'' or flowers that their thumbs can slide into. They describe the shape or feeling of rubbing during labour as ''comforting''

Womb-like, crib-like vessels remind women of opening.

A FEW PRACTICAL TIPS:

If your sculpture is solid and larger than one that can be held in the palm of your hand, scoop out the centre. Otherwise, it may explode in the kiln.

If it is hollow, make sure the walls do not vary in thickness or the heat trapped in the thickest areas will not be able to escape during firing, and your sculpture could explode in the kiln.

Pointy wing tips or finger-like projections are likely to break before or during firing. If something does break off, you can repair your sculpture with glue *after firing.*

12

Preserving Your Shape Shift: Making a Belly Cast

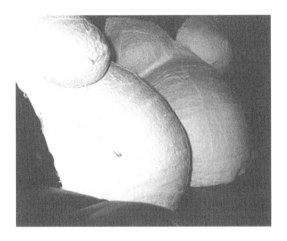

This birth art project has become a favourite at The Art of Birthing Center. You may have fun doing it, too!

In the last weeks of pregnancy (when most women are eager to escape their swollen belly and breasts), this is a wonderful way to honour and preserve the amazing reality of how your body changed to grow a baby. While making the cast, fathers often feel a new connection between themselves and the mother, and an appreciation, if not awe, of her changing body.

A photo captures your body's changes two dimensionally, but a belly cast adds the dramatic third dimension of depth. In the years to come, you can view it from all angles, touch the curves, and explore the inner concavity where your baby curled up waiting to be born.

Even if you're uncertain about doing this kind of birth art, do it anyway. As time goes by, and your love for your baby grows, this memento will mean even more to you.

MOTHER: CHOOSE YOUR POSE

STANDING, OR SITTING ON THE EDGE OF A SEAT, will result in a round, more full-bodied sculpture. Experiment with various poses: lean forward, to one side or back, or against the wall—find the shape/pose you want to preserve. Assume a position in which you can remain fairly still for about 20 minutes. DON'T LIE DOWN *(this position produces a flattened breast-belly sculpture)*.

WHAT YOU WILL NEED:

- Oil, water-soluble jelly and/or a thin layer of cotton quilt batting or cotton pre-casting padding (used to wrap a fractured extremity before casting; can be bought at a medical supply store).
- Fast-drying (5–8 minutes) plaster bandages (used to make casts for broken bones, they're inexpensive and can be bought at medical supply stores). Get eight (2 or 3 inch) rolls to cast just breast and belly, or 12 rolls if you include shoulders, upper arms and upper ⅓ of thighs. If you buy 4 or 6 inch rolls, use less.
- Plastic tablecloth, old shower curtain or a drop cloth to protect the floor.
- A cake pan of hot water—to dip strips of plaster bandages in.
- Art supplies to decorate body cast:
  Plaster of Paris: if you want to smooth the original rough gauze surface; and to enhance features such as nipples or belly button, as well as strengthen the cast.
  Wire mesh "sandpaper" to get a really smooth plaster surface.
  Gesso, paint, coloured tissue paper, feathers, beads, pictures or photos to collage, and so on.
  Shellac to seal and preserve your creation.

MAKING THE CAST

1. Fill the pan with warm water.
2. Glide *one plaster strip at a time* through the water for a few seconds. Never let go of the strip, keeping it taut, open and flat (DON'T LET IT FOLD OR TWIST ON ITSELF)
3. With the short (6 inch) strips you can gently squeeze out excess water by running your index and middle fingers down the strip.
4. Apply the strip to the mother's body. Smoothing and overlapping the strips in various directions strengthens the body cast.
5. WORK QUICKLY because the plaster begins to set (dry), and the cast begins to separate from her body about 10–15 minutes after you begin.
6. The cast will be ready to remove about five minutes after you are finished casting. Have the mother help loosen it further by doing a little "belly dance" to help loosen the cast as you ease it off at the edges.

WHAT TO DO

GETTING READY

Sculptor:
1. Put on old clothes or an apron and roll up your sleeves. You might want to take off jewellery.
2. Cover the floor with a drop cloth. Make sure room is warm but well ventilated.
3. Cut the plaster bandages into strips approximately 6, 10 and 14 inches long.
4. Generously apply lubricant to the mother's breast, belly (neck/arms/thighs), going *no more than half way* around her sides and just above the pubic hair. If necessary, use cotton padding to cover armpit, belly or pubic hair. (If you don't use enough lubrication or padding, remind the mother to use one of the pain techniques as her hair is being pulled out when the cast comes off!)

FINISHING TOUCHES

The body cast will need 48 hours to dry completely before you begin decorating it. (If it's not thoroughly dry before you seal the outside with gesso, paint or shellac, the inner layers may begin to mold.)

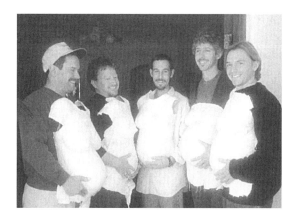

Before painting or decorating, smooth the surface of the cast by dry-walling it with a pasty mixture of plaster of Paris or paint it with gesso. (Gesso is a white, durable paint-like mixture of plaster used to prepare and smooth the surface of a sculpture before painting.)

There's no end to the decorating possibilities: paint, collage with your baby's photos or magazine cut-outs, tissue paper designs, dried flowers, beads, feathers, or written messages.

After your baby is born, you can add footprints (right where he/she used to kick you under the ribs) on the sculpture with ink or paint, …or make an impression of the footprint in wet plaster on the cast.

When you are finished, you can seal the colours and artwork with shellac.

HAVE A "CAST PARTY"

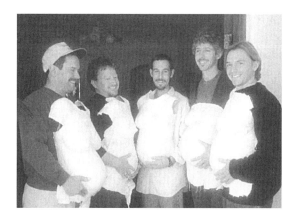

Some of my childbirth classes have had a "cast party." Each couple makes its cast in the privacy of one of the offices at the Art of Birthing Center. After sculpting, everyone proudly displays their cast with a mixture of fun and fascination as they compare all the different shapes.

While some fathers joke about using the breast and belly cast for chips'n dip, one couple had a different inspiration …

Lined with a lambskin, their belly cast became a perfect cradle for their baby's first day.

13

Birth Art Insights from Professional Artists

As the birthing from within classes evolved, my conviction grew that making birth art was a vital addition to helping women prepare for birth. I became curious what professional artists would say about the process of making and using birth art in childbirth preparation. I talked with three artists representing distinctly different, but richly rewarding perspectives.

LEAH LEE

I first saw Leah's stunning pregnant women sculptures at an exhibit. Leah, an artist and mother of two, used art to prepare for her births in the 1970's.

P.E.: What inspired you to use art as part of your preparation for birth?

LEAH: Art was so much a part of me, there was no way I couldn't. Being pregnant was the most miraculous thing that had ever happened to me. Such a wonder, such a miracle … it was a wonderful thing to express through art.

Making art during pregnancy helped me document who I was, and how I felt; what I was excited about; what I looked like—it was a way of holding that precious experience.

*

P.E.: How did you see yourself?

LEAH: I had this feeling pregnant women were out of the normal. We were attached to the earth and yet, we were floating in a kind of spiritual experience, a universal experience. There was something really special about pregnancy that made me connected to spirit in a much different way.

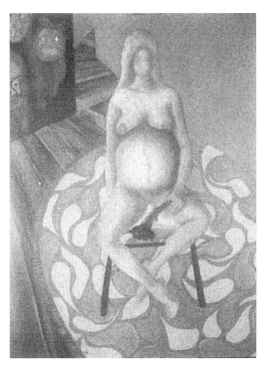

FIGURE 13.1 *Paisley Woman* by Leah Lee

*

P.E.: Did your birth art help you through labour?

LEAH: The *Paisley Woman* (Figure 13.1) got me through labour. I painted her when I was very pregnant, three-and-a-half weeks overdue according to their calculations. I don't know if they made a mistake, but I certainly *felt* 3½ weeks overdue. I was huge (laughter)!

One night I couldn't sleep, so I got up at three in the morning. I looked in the mirror and I was just blown away that I was all boobs and belly. "How did *this* happen?"

I began painting the last pregnancy self-portrait. It was a bright magenta woman with a paisley rug wrapped around her like sperm swimming around the ovum of my body … it was wonderful! There

I was in a square doorway, pushing the edges of the doorway, pushing the edges of the canvas.

I brought this painting to the hospital with me and put it where I could see it … just focusing on this picture through contractions helped a lot. With my breathing, the paisley seemed to actually move and pulse.

It must have bothered the nurse though. I remember she came in to check on me, and as she was leaving, she turned the picture around so it faced the wall! I don't know why she did that … maybe she was uncomfortable with a nude pregnant form, but, being in transition I was direct and rather forceful in having her immediately turn it around again. That picture *got* me through labour.

*

P.E.: Did anything come up in your art that was surprising?
LEAH: Oh yes! A lot. Making paintings and collages made me think and feel about being pregnant in a symbolic way, a visual way.

Six months after my baby was born, I spent a year in England, where I continued to make birth art. I had a gardener who was 80 years old and he was a very nice person, a very sweet, baroque Englishman. He wanted to model for me so I did a sculpture of his head and chest, a bust.

One day he said, "I would pose for you in the all together [nude], you know, just to help you out." When I looked at his body I realized he had a giant belly. He was mostly belly like I was in my pregnancy photographs.

So I took some photos of him and juxtaposed them with my [self-] photographs in several arrangements. This piece (Figure 13.2) evolved as a circle of life: a young woman in full bloom and a very old man in the autumn of his life. Both looking very much alike.

I pulled this shade down over their heads so you couldn't see their faces … at first glance they look like a mirror image.

Then one realizes, "Hey, wait a minute, that's an old man and she's a young woman." Hmmm … It makes one ponder a bit.

Until then all of my paintings were on rectangular canvas. But, pregnancy and birth would not work on squares. I couldn't make them work in any graceful, rhythmic, balanced or harmonious way. A circle was needed—that's what life is, a circle. I made my own circular canvases—which are quite difficult to make, taking a lot of time.

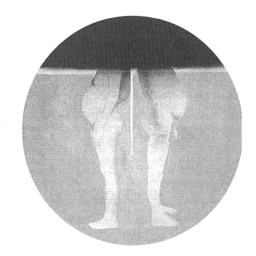

FIGURE 13.2 *Circle of Life*
by Leah Lee

*

P.E.: What advice would you give a woman hesitant to use art to help her prepare for her journey through birth?

LEAH: In some cultures there's no word for artist. Everybody has that innate urge to create, everybody is a creative being, that's human. We can't live in fear of saying our truth. What better time [to do it] then when we're so full.

The Balinese, who have no word for art, say of their art, "We have no art, we do everything as well as we can." But in our culture ... we are constricted and told from a very early age that some people are special—*they're* artists.

I used to teach art. I saw how kids' art can deteriorate from kindergarten to first, to second, to third grade. You could see it going downhill. There's a song, I can't remember who did it, "Trees are green and flowers are red. And any other way you want to do it is wrong."

There are no wrong ways to express yourself with art, but teachers want your art to be happy. "Make it pretty," they say. But, artwork isn't always pretty, sometimes it's disturbing.

You have to be very strong to be able to put out what you really feel, even when it's not culturally acceptable. Risk-taking is empowering. You don't have to put it out there [in public]. The process is very personal and the growth can be profound.

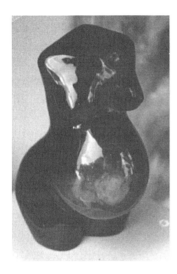

Vessel by Leah Lee

*

P.E.: What kind of response have you gotten when showing your birth art?

LEAH: People's reactions are fascinating. There always are a few positive reactions, and many embarrassed reactions. Many people are disgusted, saying, "I can't believe she would do that" or "That's disgusting, that's repulsive."

I think those reactions are a sign of fear about our bodies, about ourselves—fear of being naked, of not being pretty, not being fully clothed with our masks on.

The Venus of Willendorf torsos seem to be accepted by more people. They don't have any heads. They don't have any legs, they can't walk anywhere. They are clearly torsos, art *a la greco*. If you put faces, add hair, put vaginal lips—people freak out!

MEINRAD CRAIGHEAD

Meinrad Craighead was a Catholic nun for fourteen years before she decided to leave the convent to pursue her calling as an artist. When Meinrad came to New Mexico, she realized she had "found the land which matched my interior landscape … What my eyes saw meshed

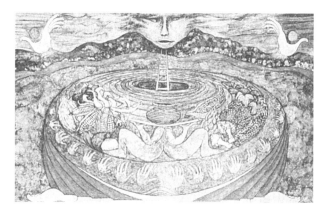

FIGURE 13.3 *Vessel* by Meinrad Craighead

with images I carried inside my body. Pictures painted on the walls of my womb began to emerge (Figure 13.3)."[1]

As an artist, Meinrad Craighead draws and paints from imagery arising from her inner life. "Each painting I make," she explains, "begins from some deep source where my mother and grandmother, and all my foremothers, still live; it is as if the line moving from pen or brush coils back to that original [place]."[2]

*

P.E.: How do the images you paint come to you?

MEINRAD: I never know what images are gestating inside of me. Some images come from dreams or daydreams. But in about a third of my drawings, I start by moving the ink or paint around on my canvas, releasing energy which has just been stored forever.

I'm not in control of the content at all, until the end, where there's a technical control needed to define and clarify the final shapes.

You can tell how important they [images] are because of the amount of energy they create for you. It's like you've been plugged into some source; your breathing rate changes, everything about you … has received something great. Something *other* has come into you, you are a receptacle for it, and become charged with this energy.

*

What you see in Meinrad's finished paintings is a mosaic composed of images coming from different layers, which had been part of each painting's development over several weeks.

Meinrad's painting process is unique. She described how she creates her paintings:

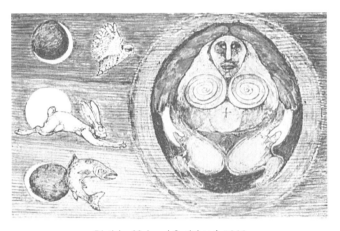

Birth by Meinrad Craighead, 1986

*

MEINRAD: I don't do any sketching. I just paint. I'm afraid sketching would dilute the power, diffuse the power. All the images in my paintings are layered. You can't identify the layers, but you can feel them ...

The final painting you see is only the surface of many things that have happened [on the canvas] in that month. Animals have come in and out, people have come in and out, whole landscapes have changed—that's all in the painting—even though you don't see it.

So every painting has its own life history—just the way you are a life history. I see only the front of you when you walk through the door, but your whole history follows invisibly behind you.

JUDY ROMINGER

Judy Rominger remembers how making birth art was an important part of her pregnancy. Judy is an art therapist in private practice and a member of the adjunct faculty in the University of New Mexico Art Therapy Program.

P.E.: How would you encourage women to prepare for birth?
JUDY: Make art, sing and dance, write and make music. Be with the earth. Spend a lot of time out in Nature. The soul just loves all this—mother soul and baby soul.

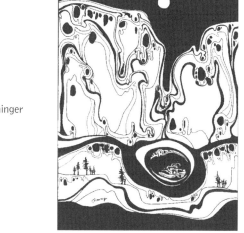

Puerta de Luna by Judy Rominger

*

P.E.: What advice would you give a woman wanting to use art as part of her preparation for childbirth?
JUDY: In my work, I encourage women to make art around any issues they're working on. For pregnant women, making art can help them find the power and support they'll need to carry them through the pregnancy, the delivery and the learning to mother.

I remember the Goddess from Mexico … [Figure 13.4, a clay sculpture of a pregnant woman giving birth squatting down, with teeth bared.] To have images like that from the imaginations of other cultures, as well as from one's own culture and one's own imagination, connects a woman to other women so that she doesn't feel so isolated in the whole mothering experience.

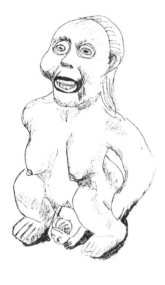

FIGURE 13.4 *Tlazaolteotl, Aztec Birth Goddess*

*

P.E.: Suppose a woman is reluctant or self-conscious about making birth art; what would you say to her?

JUDY: In our society, once a person gets out of second grade, there isn't much permission to make art unless it has been determined by someone other than yourself that you have the potential to become a *real* artist. So it's hard for us to allow ourselves to find the artist within, to value art and to value our own art-making ability.

I tell clients, "It's not about being good enough or about being a professional artist. It's about finding the images within your imagination, your soul, and then loving and honoring them by painting or sculpting or drawing them into creation. Bring your images into the world as you would bring a child into the world."

P.E.: What medium do you encourage women to use?

JUDY: In art therapy we say "the image knows what it wants." One image may want something gooey like fingerpaint, another something dry and soft like pastels, or one may call for something smooth and round like a lump of clay. So trust your intuition—whatever you feel is right for your art *is* right.

WHERE DID ALL THE BIRTH ART GO?

Beginning in the Middle Ages, women in the West were restricted from education, the practice of midwifery and medicine, and artistic expression. Even later, when active repression ended and the patriarchy "permitted" women to read and write, they had been devalued so long that they had come to believe that their lives were not worth painting or writing about.

JUDY CHICAGO

Judy Chicago is a feminist artist best known for *The Dinner Party* and *The Birth Project*. When Chicago began *The Birth Project* in 1980, she went to the library to see what images of birth she could find. She was "struck dumb" when her research "turned up almost none ... It was obvious that birth was a universal human experience and one that is central to women's lives. Why then were there no images?"[3]

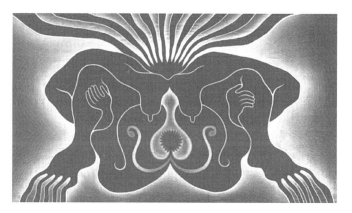

The Crowning © Judy Chicago, 1985 Needlework by Susan MacMillan, Janis Wicks, Maggie Eoyang, and Jeanette Russell

In an effort to express the "different aspects of this universal experience, the mythical, the celebratory, and the painful,"[4] Chicago spent five years designing and coordinating *The Birth Project*. This collection consists of about a hundred childbirth images realized in fabric through needlework, applique, quilting, embroidery, beadwork, and batik. All work was done in the homes of women in the United States, Canada, and New Zealand.

Preparing Your Birth Place

Chapter 14

Ask Questions Before *Your Chile Is Roasted*

When autumn comes to New Mexico, the aroma of green chile being roasted fills the air. Locals buy big burlap sacks of chile which are poured into a big drum that turns over a fire until the chile is charred (which then allows the skin to be peeled off).

Chile is mild, medium, hot, or very hot!! Locals know enough to ask, "How hot is your chile?"

One day a newcomer to New Mexico stopped at the Grocery Emporium on Girard Boulevard and bought a bag of roasted chile. The aroma made her mouth water all the way home. Using her chile, she prepared a traditional New Mexican dinner. A few bites into the meal, her eyes began to water and her tongue burned painfully.

The following day she marched up to the chile roaster and began complaining that the chile he sold her was too hot. "Look lady," he replied, "I just roast and sell chile. If you don't like your chile hot, you should've asked me about it."

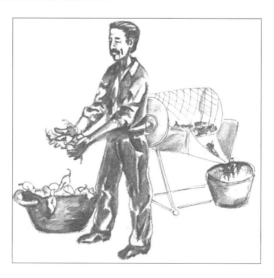

*

Like the chile customer, you need to ask your birth attendant *exactly* what he/she is selling. Birth attendants and hospitals sell a "product" day in and day out. It's your responsibility to learn more about their product (philosophy and services), and decide whether or not you want to wind up with a bag of it.

Some people put medical professionals on a pedestal, and give up taking active responsibility for their own health care. If we do not participate in decision-making, we shouldn't blame doctors or the medical establishment when things don't turn out the way we had hoped.

Doctors and midwives know a great deal about childbirth, but their knowledge has limitations, one of which is its externally-oriented objectivity. Even with their experience and good intentions, their judgement is not perfect. It's important to remember that as mothers we have exclusive access to vital information about what is happening in our bodies. Ideally, both kinds of knowing (objective and subjective) are utilized in decision-making.

*

Whether you're birthing at home or in the hospital, interviewing and selecting your birth attendant (BA) is your first step.

If a BA comes highly recommended to you by a friend, find out *specifically* what it was about their relationship she liked. In what ways were her expectations and needs met? Or not met? Most importantly, find out what your friend's expectations were in the first place. Maybe your friend wanted an episiotomy, and this particular BA performs episiotomy routinely. It was a match, and therefore your friend was satisfied with her BA.

Assessing your compatibility with a prospective birth attendant is much like the process of sorting through prospective roommates. Before moving in, you would want to reduce chances of a mis-fit by asking questions and comparing expectations and life styles.

Unfortunately, after making a first appointment with a care-giver, many women and couples act as if their responsibility in the selection process has ended. Before you jump onto the examination table, you should have a conversation clarifying what his/her methods, practices and philosophy are, and what is allowed and expected of you.

ASKING THE RIGHT QUESTIONS

Ask open-ended questions rather than questions which suggest the answer that you're looking for. Rather than inquiring, "I don't want an episiotomy. Do you cut episiotomy routinely?," ask "How many of your patients require episiotomy?" or "How do you help mums avoid tearing or episiotomy?"

If your BA answers a question about a particular procedure with "I only do that when it is necessary," consider that an inadequate response. Your next question should be, "How often do you find it necessary?"

DO YOUR EXPECTATIONS MATCH?

You are choosing a professional as a guide to help you birth normally and safely. Besides seeking professional competence and experience, you should notice whether or not this individual is a good listener and respects your ideas and questions. Pay close attention to whether he/she makes decisions *with* you, or *without* you. This is a preview of what you will likely encounter in labour.

In the UK, when you become pregnant you will be referred by your GP to a hospital and midwife service. You may be able to choose between maternity hospitals in your area, depending on where you live. In the NHS there is no guaranteed continuity of care with one practitioner; midwives usually work in teams, and a mother will see whoever is on call for her prenatal appointments and in labour.

So, if you were assuming that the person attending your birth would be the same one you'd become comfortable with during prenatal care, you may be disappointed. In any case, you need to know whether your wishes are going to be respected by others in the team-practice. It's a mistake to assume that people who work together necessarily think alike, or will honour agreements made by you with their associates. Alternatively, you may wish to consider hiring an independent midwife who can offer you continuity of care throughout pregnancy and birth, and with whom you can develop a relationship.

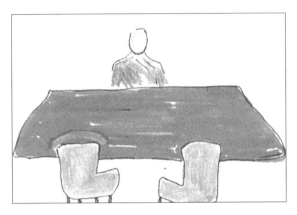

"It's hard to think about talking to my doctor about my questions. He talks down to me in the office where he sits behind his desk, an enormous desk."

THE PRENATAL COURTSHIP

Much like in the early stages of courtship, important questions and concerns may be glossed over as you're getting to know your birth attendant. Typically mothers wish to avoid risking conflict with their BA. As a result, they postpone asking hard, specific questions, until birth is staring them in the face.

That's not a good time to discover substantial differences between you and your BA. You'll feel vulnerable about confronting or leaving your BA after a relationship has developed over several months. If you do stay after a confrontation, you may fear that defensiveness or anger will linger.

Don't kid yourself. The *first* appointment is when the hard questions need to be asked and answered. Otherwise it would be like marrying someone you've met on a blind date, and learning about their beliefs and values later on.

USE YOUR POWERS OF OBSERVATION

Notice whether your BA puts you on equal or unequal footing during your prenatal visits. Here are some things to expect when you are meeting as equals:

- Meeting your BA for the first time, you should *both* be fully dressed (it's hard to pursue your questions assertively while holding a skimpy gown together).
- The BA offers or agrees to defer the complete physical until the second visit, when he/she is no longer a total stranger—and you have actually *chosen* him or her.
- Being called by your name, and not "Sweetie," "Honey," "Mum," or referred to as a medical condition (e.g., "the anaemic in room two").
- Your BA openly answers your questions about philosophy of practice and intervention statistics, such as episiotomy or Caesarean rates.
- Your BA welcomes a dialogue about how you will work together in labour and birth.

> While looking for a back-up doctor, we interviewed several doctors. I asked one, "How do you feel about me birthing in an upright or hands-and-knees position?" He rubbed his chin for a moment and said, "I used to be a vet for eight years before I became a doctor, I've done horses and cows that way, but I've never done a woman that way ... but I suppose it would be all right," he chuckled.
>
> I was surprised and appalled by his response. Rob tried to cheer me up, saying, "It's okay honey, I'll just pin a tail on you so he'll be oriented." Although in the end the doctor tried to be agreeable, we read a different message between the lines.

If later you discover that your early meetings gave you a false impression of what working with this BA would be like, you have some options:

- Attempt to communicate what's concerning you. How your BA responds is further data about whether this relationship is salvageable.
- If your gut feeling is that this BA is placating or patronizing you, choose another BA.

Remember, asking questions before your chile is roasted can save you a lot of pain in the long run.

Chapter 15

Where Mothers Build Their Nests

> Although pregnancy and birth is a richly intuitive and
> instinctive process, a woman will prepare her "nest" and birth
> according to the style of her culture, in the same way that a
> particular species of bird will build its nest with whatever is
> available.

If you envision giving birth in only one way and one place, your
chance of being thrown off balance by the unexpected increases dramatically. The more ways you can envision yourself giving birth, the
more power you bring to your own birth.

When you think about it, women give birth every day in unbelievable places and circumstances. Even as you read this, babies are
being born …

> in hot tubs, and warm ocean pools …
> in rice paddies, mountain villages, and igloos …
> in beds, birth huts, and birthing chairs.
>
> Mothers the world over give birth
> counting stars and under bright lights …
> in fields, dugouts, and by fireplaces …
> in planes and trains …
> in one-room shacks and operating rooms.
>
> Mothers and nature always find a way.

Even when a woman believes *she* has chosen her birth place, there are
unseen, powerful forces narrowing the parameters within which she
has chosen. Adrienne Rich, author of *Of Women Born*, observed,
"One does not give birth in a void, but rather in a cultural and

political context. Laws, professional codes, religious sanctions, and ethnic traditions all affect a woman's choices concerning childbirth."[1]

In reality, not many women or couples freely choose their birth place. Sometimes it is an eager baby who "decides" where it will be born. More often these days it is health insurance which most influences where we give birth.

NETSILIK ESKIMO BIRTH

"She brings her child into the world while on her knees and alone, without help. If it is winter, she allows the child to glide down into a small hollow in the snow on the platform itself. No skin lining is placed in the hollow for the child, which falls straight into the snow."

– RASMUSSEN, AN ANTHROPOLOGIST, 1931[3]

BIRTH COCOONS

One of the most difficult things for a mother to come to terms with is that she cannot predict or control her birth or birth environment. Fortunately, it's not just the birth *place* that makes your birth memorable or powerful, it's you and what you bring to it. Even if birth attendants seem busy or hurried, and the environment clinical or impersonal, it's still possible for you to spin an insulating cocoon of love and warmth around each other as you bring your baby into the world.

Do what you need to do to make your birth easier. For example, Anastasia, a wonderful labour and delivery nurse, told me about a first-time, strong-bodied, strong-minded mother who had impressed her by how she'd made the hospital birth space her own.

This mum arrived in active labour with her huge inflated blue physiotherapy ball … She got on her ball and wouldn't get off it until it was nearly time to deliver. She knew what she wanted and needed, and she got it. She did not want to be touched or disturbed until it was time to push. Labour took a long time, and near the end she was running out of energy. Her nurse-midwife explained to her that she needed more energy to finish labour and to push out the baby and suggested an IV. The woman didn't "want" an IV, but she wanted to give birth and accepted it. The IV did re-energize her and she gave birth shortly afterwards.

It might be your nurse or birth attendant who is the one to spin a cocoon of love around you, as was the case of the midwife who spent the day labouring with Kianna, a first-time mother. It just so happened that Kianna became completely dilated and ready to push just as the nursing shifts were changing. Kianna had been labouring in a small labour room and policy required that she be moved down the hall (past the crowded and noisy nurses' station) to a birthing room.

> "A !Kung mother takes great pride in self-sufficiency in birth. As soon as her contractions become strong, the mother goes out in the veld. She collects soft grass and piles it into a mound to make a soft landing for her baby. When pushing, she squats over that mound.
>
> During her first labour, her mother and other older women assist her. If the first birth goes well, she will give birth to subsequent babies alone. If labour begins at night, she will not wake her sleeping husband as she slips out the door and goes to the veld. !Kung mothers have a keen sense of competence and independence. In the morning, the !Kung mother, glowing with pride, returns home with her newly born child."[3]

Kianna's nurse helped protect her concentration by whispering encouraging words in her ear, saying things like "These are really bright lights, stay where you're at … There are people working at the desk, stay inside yourself … " until they arrived in the privacy of the birth room. Forty minutes later Kianna gave birth to her baby girl.

Judy Graham describes how she and Michel Odent (renowned French obstetrician and author of the instant classic, *Birth Reborn*) chose their birthplace. Judy shared her story in *Nursing Times* (1977):

What I wanted was a place where I could feel uninhibited; where I could be free during labour and birth to adopt any position I wanted—when I wanted; where there would be no unnecessary medical interference; where I could have complete privacy; where I could be alone with my partner; where there would be no strangers observing me and watching the clock. It had to be a place where I could give birth wherever my instincts told me was right; where I would not be moved from place to place each time I reached a new stage of labour. It had to have the right atmosphere, with dim lights or even darkness; no hustle and bustle, nor rules and regulations, and no hospital policies. And it had to be somewhere where we would be left undisturbed with the newborn baby for as long as we wanted.

REASSURANCE OR DISTRACTION: MUMS' REACTIONS TO FOETAL MONITOR

In one study (Starkman, 1976) of twenty-five mothers' reactions to the foetal monitor, the nine who had experienced a previous stillbirth or infant death felt positively about the foetal monitor. The constant sound representing baby's heart beat was especially reassuring to this group.

Twelve mothers saw the monitor as an extension of the physician, providing reassurance and protection to them and their babies. Others saw it as an extension of themselves, providing accurate information to the physician, and relieving them of that responsibility.

Ten of the fifteen mothers who had no history of pregnancy loss had negative reactions to foetal monitoring. Some mothers felt the monitor distracted their husband's and doctor's attention away from them. Seven complained of increased discomfort, especially with the insertion of internal catheters.

Eight complained of enforced immobility. Several complained about the "hustle and bustle and lack of privacy caused by extra people coming in to fix the monitor" (when it was having mechanical difficulties); and about "the buzzing and clicking, especially when they felt out of control." Others were frightened by any slowing of the foetal heart rate."

I doubt that there's a hospital the length and breadth of Britain where a woman can have all this!

By contrast, my own home had everything we needed. And the more I considered hospital delivery suites, the more I was convinced that my house was much better suited to our particular needs.

Another reason why home birth was really the only choice open to us was because any hospital would have classified me as high risk and felt that routine intervention was justified. I was 38, having a first baby and had been diagnosed as having multiple sclerosis 11 years ago. On top of that, my blood pressure has always been high.

Michel strongly believes that the higher risk the woman is, the less she should be disturbed while giving birth. ... As for the birth. It was fast and easy—the midwives arrived only just in time. My labour was only three hours from first contraction to delivery, with no complications.[4]

Judy and Michel's needs were met by staying at home, but other couples' needs might be met in a birth centre or hospital. Some mothers (and fathers) feel reassured by technological support and choose to birth in a hospital. In addition, many hospitals are working toward making their environment less clinical and more home-like; some also offer nurse-midwifery services.

So, as part of making your choice of birth place a conscious decision, challenge your assumptions and allow your imagination to consider a range of possible settings.

Chapter 16

Childbirth As a Rite of Passage

Birth profoundly changes people—socially, spiritually and psychologically. All who participate in birth, not just mothers, are affected by its power. Yet our culture seems to have forgotten this.

When I learned about the ways elders and shamans traditionally have used rituals to celebrate major life transitions, I became excited thinking about what the "ritual" of childbirth classes could offer women.

Realizing how hungry women are for guidance from older, experienced women, I no longer want to limit my role to just "teacher." Expectant mothers need to be mothered; their hearts need to be infused with love, confidence, and determination.

I now see myself as a "midwife" to the gestation and birth of women as mothers. I've also come to realize that *any* childbirth preparation inevitably becomes a transition ritual, for better or worse.

THE HYPNOTIC POWER OF RITUAL AND SYMBOLS

Birth is a universal experience, but the rituals surrounding it are remarkably different across cultures and over time. Traditional birth rituals offer inspiration, illumination and group support. In the West, however, there are few birth rituals that work that way. What we do have are medical birth customs rich with symbols (although their significance usually goes unnoticed).

A ritual is any message that is repetitively and non-verbally communicated in order to bring the behaviour and values of its recipients into alignment with the sender's. *Routine* obstetric care, by delivering the same message again and again to women and families, constitutes a ritual.

Rituals send messages through symbols and symbolic behaviour. Symbols communicate in a uniquely effective way because they, unlike the written word, are received unexamined and unquestioned by the right brain, where they are felt *instantly* throughout the body-mind.

> What feelings and mindset are evoked in you by symbols like the American flag or a crucifix?

OBSTETRIC SYMBOLS

Consider the symbols commonly found in a clinical birth place, such as the clock on the wall, the foetal monitor, stirrups, hospital beds, gowns and masks, IV's or the patient ID wristband. Similarly, a home birth has its own set of symbols, like a familiar bed and cozy surroundings, pets, back yard, photos, and the aroma of food cooking in the kitchen.

In my classes I ask parents to list every obstetric symbol they can think of. Then we take a look at the messages those symbols send. For example, when the foetal monitor is viewed as an *obstetric symbol*, something dramatic happens. Parents realize for the first time how that "symbol" indirectly but powerfully communicates the potential for crisis. That message affects their feelings, expectations and behaviours (along with everyone else's). This new awareness usually leads to a lively discussion of how obstetric symbols influence labour.

Let's take a look at another example of an obstetric symbol: the hospital gown (it's not just a grotesque fashion statement!). As you look at this illustration ask yourself:

- What symbolic messages are communicated by this picture?
- What is your immediate visceral or emotional reaction?
- What role and behaviours does the symbol of the hospital gown hypnotically suggest?
- How might wearing this gown affect how you will act in labour?

The hospital gown is just another example; keep in mind that every thing and every person (including you) involved in a ritual sends a message to the unconscious. This includes your doctor, midwife and nurse, who not only send messages, but receive them as well. A father in one of my childbirth classes, an emergency room doctor, explained how walking into a cubicle and seeing a patient lying down in a hospital gown affects his perception. And how differently he views that same person a few minutes later when he/she is dressed and upright.

*

If you are birthing in a hospital, I suggest you bring your symbols to decorate your birth room:

- *Bring* your own pillow, the sculpture you made, and a bouquet of flowers.
- *Hang* your own artwork, that you made, or find inspirational; or photographs of babies.
- *Wear* your own t-shirt.
- *Play* your own music.

FINDING NEW MEANINGS

Julia Knight-Williamson, a midwife, told me about a diabetic mother whose birth needed to be medically managed in the hospital. However, this mother was creative in the way she gave obstetric symbols new meaning: instead of viewing the IV as a symbol of restraint, she decided to see her IV pole as a "tree of life" nourishing her in labour. This positive perception helped her embrace her birth in the way it needed to happen.

DRAWING ON OUR BIRTH CUSTOMS

To help mothers learn more about how they have internalized our birth customs and routine practices, I ask them to draw an Artist-Historian picture:

IMAGINE YOU ARE AN ARTIST-HISTORIAN SHOWING SOMEONE FROM ANOTHER PLANET OR CULTURE WHAT BIRTH IN OUR CULTURE IS LIKE. YOUR ASSIGNMENT

IS TO RECORD IN A DRAWING, OR A SERIES OF DRAWINGS, HOW WOMEN GIVE BIRTH IN THIS TIME AND PLACE.

DRAW THE BIRTH PLACE AND ILLUSTRATE THE CUSTOMS. IF THERE ARE PEOPLE, SHOW WHAT THEY ARE DOING THERE. TRY TO BE OBJECTIVE. THIS MAY OR MAY NOT REPRESENT YOUR OWN BIRTH EXPECTATIONS OR VALUES, BUT IT SHOULD REPRESENT THE CURRENT BIRTH CUSTOMS.

In the three examples that follow, you will see the rich material this assignment brings up. Often mothers do not even know they feel apprehensive about being in a hospital until they make, and contemplate, this drawing. Bringing their anxiety to conscious awareness allows time to investigate and tour the hospital, prepare their birth space, face reality and dispel myths.

TRY THIS:

1. Divide a sheet of paper into three columns.
2. In the first column, list every birth symbol you can think of.
3. Next to this list, write the meaning you associate with it.
4. In the last column, assign a new meaning. It might be a more positive or objective meaning, but it could also be a negative one. This is a way of transcending your assumptions of what particular symbols communicate.

In the first drawing, done in light blue crayon (Figure 16.1), a first-time mother who said she had never seen a birth, or talked with anyone about their birth experience, drew this image. She commented that she really didn't know where it came from, but it was her first and strongest image.

Don't make the mistake of dismissing this drawing just because the antiquated custom of holding a newborn baby upside down and making it cry has been abandoned. For this mum, the value of a drawing like this was the discussion that followed. It opened the door to discovering her feelings of isolation, anxiety about being able to protect her baby, and personal insignificance in the event.

Look at the drawing and listen to what she has to say:

I used blue on white to represent sterile and the blue clothes they wear. The lights are big huge, silver lights—give a white feeling. The baby being held upside down is being made to cry. The mother is there, kind of, but she's not the focus. The father's not around—the mother disappears into the background.

I wanted this drawing to be stark, so I did not put an expression on the baby or doctor. Every woman will have a different experience or reaction, but these routine events will happen many times. I didn't want an umbilical cord attached, I wanted the mother to feel like she's barely there.

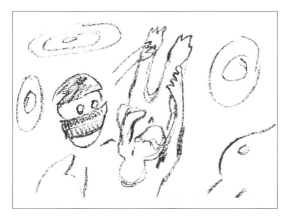

FIGURE 16.1 A mother encounters her unspoken fears of isolation and personal insignificance in her *Artist-Historian* drawing.

*

Here's another example of an *Artist-Historian* drawing, and what the mother said about it:

This [picture] (Fig. 16.2) is a portrayal of hospital birth, the way some babies are born. Mothers [grey bodies] are not individuals, but seen as a herd of mothers. The idea is to get the baby out of them in the quickest, most efficient way possible … using equipment to accomplish that [instruments on right]. Birth is removed from the process. You are there as a specimen to be treated, worked on, handled. The object is to get the baby out of her.
Here [upper margin] is the result. Babies lying in bubbles all in rows.

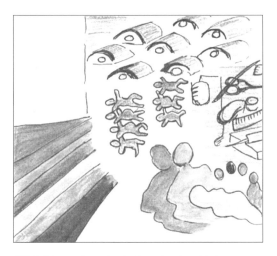

FIGURE 16.2 A mother's view of techno-birth customs.

[The colourful rainbow, lower left, is] "the vision of a terrestrial being looking down at our birth customs. The colourful family on the lower right is a family who chose to birth at home or in a birth centre.

A drawing and commentary like Figure 16.2 leads naturally to a discussion of where and how the artist-mother wants to have her birth. This mother had had two successful home births, and was planning another. Still, there's always some possibility of a hospital transfer occurring. My work with a woman like this would include preparation for birthing, even in a hospital, with integrity and emotional resiliency.

I have seen similar drawings from women who were planning to have a hospital birth. In that case the image invites an exploration of whether that decision was determined by financial, family or cultural pressures, rather than by her needs and desires.

*

The last example (Figure 16.3) was drawn by a pregnant mother (and postpartum nurse) who described her first birth, in the hospital, as fairly positive. Nevertheless, she still believed that the hospital's *primary* concern was efficiency. Her anxiety about hospitals intervening too readily is represented by her written words, "Let's just cut it out."

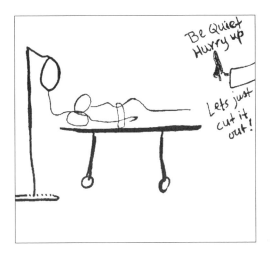

FIGURE 16.3 A mother confronts her underlying anxiety about hospitals' proclivity towards efficiency and intervention.

Even though she portrayed our birth customs this way, she didn't think this would happen to *her*. Here's what she said about her drawing:

This [picture] is not how I'm gonna do it. This mother is actually fine with this, she's uneducated, not aware that this is not helping her.

I got the "Be Quiet" at my last birth. ... "Put your knees together ... the doctor's not here yet." ... Then they got the forceps out when the doctor came. I had to push fast—and didn't get the forceps. That's the doctor's arm [on the right] with a knife. The mother was making too much noise. "Tie her down—knock her out." This birth's not natural, not normal. The doctor is saying "Be Quiet—Hurry Up" and "Let's just cut it out."

Months later, in the postpartum interview, she described her recent birth experience, and then referred back to her drawing:

I was just beginning labour, or so I thought. The mild contractions I had had all day did not seem very significant, but they must have been working. I was calmly resting in the hospital, when the contractions seemed a little stronger.

I called in the nurse, who called the doctor. He reached in without ever looking at me or speaking to me, and said, "She's eight [centimetres dilated], give me an internal foetal electrode … let's put 'er on the monitor" … he gave lots of orders.

Before I knew it they had put oxygen on me and were frowning at the monitor strip, commenting to each other about "decelerations," but no one talked to *me*, or explained anything about my baby's [heart rate] decelerations … did they think I wasn't interested? The monitor was the focus. I wasn't the focus. I was the process creating the data.

Nobody touched me except to adjust the monitor. I suddenly felt as if I were an entity containing the baby and all they cared about was the baby. I was the machine. The end product was the baby.

How could I be there and not be the focus? It was as if I wasn't even there. What I wanted didn't matter.

Later, after the baby was born, they said my baby wasn't warm enough and they took him to the nursery. I was thinking "I'm not a good mother—I can't even keep him warm."

I have been thinking about that picture I drew with you when I was pregnant … the picture of the woman with the restraints. In labour, I was *that* woman, but the restraints used on me were invisible … they made all the decisions … they kept me from participating in my own birth.

This moving story shows that even in a drawing assignment portraying the birth customs of a culture, the personal concerns of the mother-artist can be inferred from the content and mood of the drawing. Once this information is brought to the surface, the stage is set to work more deeply with a mother's emotional/psychological preparation.

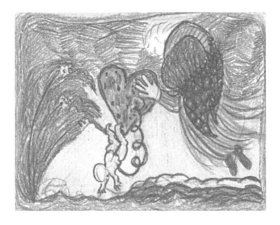

"This is a midwife's angel shaking the baby out of its mother's heart and into the sea of life. But she's got hold of the umbilical cord so that the baby won't get hurt. The plants on the left are sperm and egg plants; the baby comes "out of the blue" and into the "light."

Earth and love surround the whole thing in the border."

Midwife Elizabeth Gilmore, Taos, New Mexico

ANCESTRAL AND MODERN HEALING RITUALS

> Through knowledge, the unconscious is robbed of its fire.
>
> CARL G. JUNG

You might find it interesting to contrast the active participation required of initiates in ancestral rituals with our culture's style of "giving" education, religion and medical treatment to the passive recipient.

In some traditional societies, the applicant is not taken through the ritual just because she is of age or it is "time." She must show she is ready from the heart; she must appeal to the elders, expressing her conviction, trust, and readiness to enter into the ritual.

Ancient shamanic rituals are designed to help a person go beyond the limits of her conscious mind, where she may access healing images, visions and insights. Knowledge is not "given" to the initiate; rather she is led to the spring of her unconscious from which truth of a more personal nature will flow.

Just as a shaman cannot *give* a patient a healing vision, there are some kinds of learning a childbirth teacher can't give a mother. A knowledgeable childbirth teacher can inform mothers *about* birth, physiology, hospital policies, complications and technology. But that kind of information doesn't touch what a mother actually experiences *in* labour, or what she needs to know as a mother (not a patient) in this rite of passage.

If your job was to teach someone what chocolate tastes like, how would you do it? What would he know after you told him *about* its taste, colours, shape, texture and chemical composition. No matter how much *information* you provide, you can't give him the sensory, personal experience of chocolate.

SO, WHAT SHOULD A CHILDBIRTH TEACHER DO?

Birthing From Within recognizes the significance of traditional rituals of initiation and preparation. Its emphasis is on creating opportunities for personal learning, rather than the transmission of information. Secrets locked in mothers' hearts are discovered and shared through activities such as art, poetry, writing, freeflowing discussions, and laughter.

BIRTH CUSTOMS AND RITUALS AROUND THE WORLD

The positive intention of all birth customs and rituals, including ours, is to ensure safety of the woman through her unpredictable journey of birth. In their article, "Imagery and Symbolism in the Birth Practices of Traditional Cultures," Brian Bates and Allison Newman Turner describe the following metaphorical, religious and sexual imagery used worldwide to enhance the birthing woman's participation in her birth. Metaphorical imagery is intended to help the mother release, open up and deliver the baby.

In the Philippine islands …
it is customary to put a key (unlocking)
and a comb (untangling)
under the labouring woman's pillow;
the moultings from snakes or other animals

may be used to make a belt for the parturient woman;
… a house ladder may be turned upside down,
knives unsheathed,
recently madefurniture unnailed,
recently sewn seams ripped open and
drawers, trunks and cupboards unlocked.

In Delhi villages
all knots in clothing ropes and the woman's hair are loosened to
relieve the pain of contractions.

Also in India,
prolonged labour may be treated by
placing a tightly furled flower beside the woman
in the belief that as it unfurls
so will the woman's cervix dilate.

The Vietnamese refer to birth in terms reflecting this—
"the bud opens and the flower blooms."

The Maltese keep a flower in water in the delivery room saying
that when the bud blooms the child will be born,
and in the Philippine villages
the midwife throws a handful of flowers at the woman
in labour when she arrives at the house.[1]

To this day many customs symbolically work to "appease or distract the appropriate spirits away from the labouring woman."[2] For example, the Cuna Indians of Panama believe a difficult labour is caused by the spirit of the womb, Muu, who is holding onto the baby and not letting it out. In such cases, the midwife calls the shaman or medicine man to sing the hypnotic Cuna birth song:

The shaman sits beneath the labouring woman's hammock and sings to her in great repetitive detail the story of how and why he has been called to attend her and subsequently the attack that he and his fellow spirits are launching upon Muu's possessiveness, in order to release the baby. He describes to the woman how they enter the vagina single file and make their way up to the uterus. They call upon the aid of the souls of the other organs of the body and those of the various animals to help in the "victorious combat" with Muu. The wood-boring insects are asked to cut through the tangled fibers; the burrowing insects are called upon to help the baby move down the birth canal. As the shaman and his fellow spirits leave the vagina they march out in a [horizontal] row rather than single file, signifying that dilation is complete.[3]

Bates and Turner suggest that the shaman's song provides the labouring woman a symbolic context for her experience of pain. She is no longer labouring alone and in isolation, but in harmony with the rest of her society, placing her within a cosmic order, which connects her to nature and to her fellow beings [and other living things].

*

Every mother must find, within herself and her culture, metaphorical imagery which will uplift, inspire and help her open body-heart-and-mind in labour. Plan your own symbolic labour ritual or write yourself a birth song.

Chapter 17

The Birth Plan Trap

Writing birth plans is becoming a ritual of modern pregnancy. This practice began with the positive intention of encouraging parents to take a more active role in birth. Writing a birth plan motivates parents to learn about their hospital's routines (usually with the intention of avoiding them). A birth plan also can be a tool to open dialogue with doctors. Telling a doctor what you want (and seeing his/her reactions) allows insight into the doctor's philosophy of practice and willingness to share decision-making.

While gaining information is advantageous, the subtle implications of writing a birth plan are more complex than many people realize. If you look below the surface, you'll see that birth plans are like a hidden reef on which your efforts towards deeper birth preparation may run aground.

In my classes I discourage mothers and fathers from writing a birth plan. I've changed my mind on this issue for several reasons. I now believe that the need to write a birth plan invariably comes from:

- Anxiety and/or mistrust of the people who will be attending you;
- A natural fear of the unknown. Some women attempt to ease that fear, and enhance their sense of control, by writing a detailed script of how the birth should happen;
- Lack of confidence in self and/or birth-partner's ability to express and assert what is needed in the moment. (Birth plans may be intended to substitute for face-to-face negotiations with authority figures.)

BIRTH IS WHAT'S HAPPENING WHILE YOU'RE BUSY WRITING BIRTH PLANS

The idea of planning a birth is naive; labour and birth are not events conducive to being planned. You can have a fantasy or birth plan, the hospital has its ideas, but Mother Nature may surprise all of you.

In writing a birth plan, a woman focuses on fending off outside forces which she fears will shape her birth. This effort distracts her from trusting herself, her body, and her spirituality. Rather than planning her own hard work and surrender, her energy is diverted towards controlling the anticipated actions of others.

There are no unique birth plans. While your birth plan is unique to you, it won't seem that way to your hospital or doctor. All women ask for the same thing: respect, dignity, support to birth naturally with minimal routine intervention and no unnecessary separation from the baby.

Trying to change the medical system risks creating defensive, resistant, and hyper-vigilant mindsets. You may feel a sense of power during this process, but it's an illusion, and more importantly, a distraction from developing genuine personal power. This fear-based, externally directed preparation ("I don't want this," "I don't want that") flows unproductively through the mind-body connection; it's harder for your body to let go when your guard is up.

WHEN YOU KNOW YOUR SHIP IS "UNSINKABLE,"
YOU DON'T WORRY ABOUT ICEBERGS, OR LIFEBOATS.

Another hidden danger is when an authority "accepts" a birth plan during pregnancy. At that point, there's a strong tendency for women to stop worrying, stop exploring and stop accessing personal resources.

Chapter 18

Birthing With Wolves

Serena had her first child by Caesarean for failure to progress. She doubted she "needed" the Caesarean and suspected that factors other than her inability to birth normally contributed to her long labour.

> I had to lie flat on my back, I wasn't allowed to eat or drink, and I lost my grip when labour really hurt—I had been led to expect labour pain would feel like "squeezes." There was no experienced labour assistant to tell me what to expect or do, and the doctor yelled at me for taking him out of a Christmas party!

Pregnant with her second child, Serena was planning to birth with midwives in the hospital. She was using art therapy to help her move from passive fear to a more active role in her upcoming birth. At our last class she told me about a small drawing she had nade at home, which was to play an important role in her birth:

> An image of a wolf came to me when I was waking from a nap; a big, scruffy, sinister-looking wolf with red teeth. It seemed to be warning me to do something, saying without out words, "Open your eyes! You listen to what I say, girl."
>
> The wolf seemed to have a flame inside, it was glowing through its ears, eyes and skin [gold] … maybe it was a guide for me. It made me think of Vasalisa in *Women Who Run With the Wolves* where she is given a lighted skull as a symbol of the power she had—knowing and intuition.

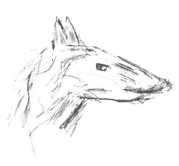

Serena's scruffy, protective wolf-guide

When I was in labour, I asked Bill [Serena's husband] to hold the wolf [drawing] in front of my face. I'd stare at it until I got the reassurance I needed, until it talked to me. Then I'd let him put it down again. It'd say, without words, it was more of a feeling, "Don't be naive. Take yourself seriously. Don't let people take care of you unless you tell them to or want them to … don't pretend to be tough when you're not."

I realized there was a paradox: when you pretend to be tough, your power is somewhere else—but sometimes when you look rattled, you're actually more alive and loose.

Serena, with help from her "inner wolf," laboured hard and fought for what she needed. She gave birth normally, in awareness, as she had known she could.

*

A SHE-WOLF IN HER DEN: REBECCA'S STORY

You can imagine how fiercely a mother wolf protects her birth space. Human mothers, however, are socialized never to growl or show their claws. Furthermore, a woman at the hospital is not on her own turf, which makes it more difficult to protect. In the hospital you are a visitor, but a woman's home is *her* territory.

Rebecca, in labour with her third child, became a "Wild Wolf" marking territory at her home in the Manzano Mountains on the outskirts of Albuquerque. When I arrived to attend her birth, Rebecca was in good labour, still actively tending to her two children. During contractions she stopped whatever she was doing, stretched and rubbed circles softly on her belly. After the contraction passed, she went on about her business.

Predicting Rebecca would birth in about two hours, I called a second midwife, Donna. A family friend came to watch the older children.

Upon Donna's arrival, Rebecca's labour pattern changed. Later she had this to say about it:

Since I hadn't met Donna before, I needed to check her out before I could give birth. I had to take her outside [the house] to protect my

birth space; I showed her the garden and we played with the dogs …
I felt like I put labour on hold for about two hours—spending this
time getting to know her. It was as though I was "sniffing out her
scent," checking out her unfamiliar presence, because I wasn't sure
how safe she was. This done, I could return to my birth place and
focus on giving birth. All this was more subconscious than conscious,
and only became clear later.

During those two hours, labour didn't stop, but it slowed down.
Suspecting Rebecca's need for privacy, I suggested Donna and I leave
for an hour and go to a nearby restaurant for lunch. Later, Rebecca,
identifying our departure as a turning point in her labour, said:

> I felt a sigh of relief to be alone. I had been entertaining, being a host-
> ess to the midwives. After the midwives left I took a shower, then laid
> down on my bed. Labour became serious about an hour later. I was
> labouring by myself in our bedroom. My husband was in the kitchen
> doing the dishes when I called to him to call the midwives back!

When we returned, Rebecca was lying on her side, with that faraway
Labourland look. The afternoon light filtered through the blinds.
When asked how she felt, Rebecca said, "I feel like a mother wolf in
her den." Indeed, she looked like a mother wolf lying on her side,
panting and pushing quietly. With her husband lying at her side, and
the children watching with quiet excitement, their daughter was born
peacefully and gently.

Privacy may be a key to birthing normally. Mammals insist on privacy to give birth, and so should you. You will be less self-conscious
and more self-aware in the privacy of your own home or labour room
(if someone's guarding the door).

Chapter 19

Home Birth

To the surprise of many of my friends, this chapter almost didn't get written. They knew I had attended home births and were puzzled how I could write a book about birth and not include a chapter on home birth. Knowing that most people are unaware of the safety of an attended home birth, I was concerned about being viewed as a professional-on-the-fringe, or discounted as someone whose personal experiences and preferences had clouded her objective judgement about birth.

As a childbirth teacher, one of my greatest challenges is to inform people objectively about their choices and give them respectful support in decision-making, so they are not left feeling coerced or guilty about whatever informed choice they eventually make. I've become increasingly concerned about the Rule of the Righteous in the Land of Birth: breastfeeding mothers who disdain those who bottlefeed; women sworn to epidurals who mock mothers pursuing natural childbirth; or doctors who accuse parents birthing at home of being irresponsible and selfish.

So, in trying to downplay my own biases, I went too far in the other direction, both in my classes and in writing this book. In an effort to be non-intrusive, I was short-changing people by withholding vital information they were unlikely to encounter elsewhere. One winter night my eyes were opened.

As the book was nearing completion (without this chapter), I was teaching a childbirth class of six couples. One of the mothers was sharing her fears about the multiple uncertainties she would encounter when she arrived in labour at the hospital. She and her husband (a physician) reported that they had been exploring the possibility of having a home birth. Two of their physician-friends had chosen home births, and had spoken positively about their experiences. Within minutes the class erupted into animated discussion, provocative questions and a sense of hopeful excitement about having an additional choice to consider.

At the end of class, five of the six couples decided to investigate home birth further. Two of the fathers gently confronted me about why my classes hadn't routinely included information about the option of home birth. Like most couples, they hadn't considered home birth because they didn't know it was still an option. They expressed concern that if the issue hadn't come up that night, they wouldn't have learned that healthy mothers don't *have* to go to the hospital; they can choose an attended birth at home instead.

At the end of class, one mother sighed with relief, "I feel more relaxed—just knowing a home birth is a possibility, whether or not I choose it."

THE PHILOSOPHICAL ASSUMPTIONS OF HOME BIRTH PARENTS AND ATTENDANTS

- Because pregnancy and birth are natural physiological events, normal birth does not belong in hospitals.
- The natural course of labour is already perfect, and should be interfered with as little as possible.
- Pain is part of an essential and healthy feedback mechanism in labour, which women can learn to cope with, with proper encouragement and support.
- Medical management of pregnancy and birth should be limited to those which are medically complicated.
- Unnecessary medical interventions complicate normal labour, creating additional risk and the need for *more* intervention.

LABOURING AT HOME

In some circles, labouring or birthing at home is considered a radical idea. Most first-time mothers I talk to doubt they know enough to give birth *anywhere*, much less at home. They are surprisingly out of touch with the innate, miraculous processes involved in giving birth. Even though those mothers don't know birth technology either, they know it's out there. Daughters of our technological age, surrounded by cellular phones and lightning-fast computers, understandably have faith in technology.

For fathers, of course, the wisdom of a mother's body is a *total* mystery. Furthermore, men have a greater tendency to admire and immerse themselves in technological "toys." That interest, when combined with well-intentioned concern about the welfare of their wife and baby, creates a strong push for a medicalized birth in the hospital (even when the mother wants to consider labouring or birthing at home).

In addition, women/couples who plan to labour at home as long as they can, or intend to birth at home, typically get little support and a lot of anxious scepticism from those around them. Under such circumstances, feeling a bit uneasy is to be expected. Still, if you know that you do not want to labour (or birth) in the hospital unnecessarily (i.e., when your midwife tells you everything is proceeding normally at home), consider the following mind-set:

The truth is nobody can pre-plan a birth; even the most adamant home birth advocates can't make it happen at home by willing it. If you sense that the privacy of your own home will make labour easier for you, but you don't want to make a commitment to *birth* at home, try a more flexible mind set: Make a commitment to *labour* at home with an experienced attendant. If labour and pushing progress normally, the baby literally will "fall out" at home. If labour does not progress easily, or you want to be in the hospital for any reason, go there.

One advantage of labouring in the privacy of your home, with one-on-one midwifery support, is that should a problem arise that requires medical support at the hospital, you will not wonder whether your labour problems were caused by routine, unnecessary, or ill-timed hospital interventions. It is also easier to accept medical interventions (at the time, and in retrospect), when a midwife, whose philosophy and practice is not centred around such interventions, has endorsed their necessity.

A TIMELY TRANSFER: WHEN A HOSPITAL IS THE PLACE TO BIRTH

Right now, birthing women in developed countries can have the best of both worlds: 1) safer home births with modern midwives trained to identify and manage minor problems, and 2) the availability, within minutes, of appropriate hospital technology if necessary.

Couples and professional midwives planning a home birth know their ultimate goal is a safe birth, not a home birth at any cost. Couples are relieved to learn that transfers to a hospital rarely involve a labour *emergency*. Most of the time problems in labour develop slowly; watchful midwives see them coming like the headlight of a train down a darkened track.

Usually transfers are for non-emergency reasons, such as a prolonged, exhausting labour, failure to progress in dilation or pushing, or too much time having elapsed after the water has broken. Typically a couple drives to the hospital (with their midwife) in their own vehicle, without needing to run any red lights. It's unusual for an ambulance or paramedics to be necessary.

Being at home also means being "at home" psychologically. Sometimes a woman planning to birth at home is unable to give birth there—but upon crossing the emergency room threshold her child is quickly born! It's reasonable that women who hold an unrecognized belief that the hospital is a safer birth place, will have difficulty letting go at home.

Couples experience many benefits from birthing at home. Nevertheless, there are rare occurrences when a birth emergency arises that would have had a better outcome in the hospital. This reality is part of what a couple needs to consider in choosing the birth setting which is best for them.

"Until the eighteenth century, women generally gave birth without any medication at all, even when their labors were complicated and required the use of forceps (invented around 1600) or the performance of cesarean section. Most people felt this was in keeping with the Bible's dictum that women should 'bring forth children in sorrow.' This so-called 'divine law' was so strictly adhered to that in sixteenth-century Edinburgh a woman was burned at the stake for having received a certain medicine for pain relief during childbirth."[1]

— SHARRON HANNON
CHILDBIRTH: A SOURCE BOOK

"BE GRATEFUL FOR EVERY LITTLE MERCY"

If you were hoping to avoid medical intervention, finding yourself in need of it can bring feelings of disappointment. However, medical technology can be viewed through different lenses. Some may see it as a confirmation of helplessness or failure; others perceive it as an ally supporting their journey through pregnancy and birth.

I will always appreciate the teaching of Sufi Master Irina Tweedie. I met her in October, 1984, when I arrived at her doorstep soaked from a London rain shower. A kindly old woman, with wispy, white hair pulled back into a small tight bun, invited me in. Her unforgettable, translucent, watery-blue eyes and tranquil countenance told me without asking, who she was.

The house was full of people from all over the world who had come to study the Sufi path and meditate with her. During one of our visits, Mrs. Tweedie was marveling at a news story describing how medical technology miraculously had saved a life. She said softly, "Modern medicine is a miracle, a wonderful miracle. Each of us should be mindful of our blessed karma to be born in this time, so that if we need a wonder drug or specialized surgical technique, we can have it. We should be humble and grateful to live in the countries where such help is available. Be grateful for every little mercy."

HOME BIRTH ECONOMICS

Legally, home birth in the UK is covered by the NHS. However, hospitals may tell the labouring mother, on the day she calls in, that there are no midwives to attend her at home so she'll have to come in to the hospital. A way of avoiding this is to hire an independent midwife who can ensure continuity of care throughout pregnancy, birth and postpartum. More and more women are choosing this option. The fees may range from £1,000 to £4,000, depending on the area you live in and the services which they provide. Some will allow you to pay in instalments. Occasionally it is possible for your GP to refer you to independent midwives, and to use the GP's practice funds to pay for your care.

*

Studying the economics of birth in other developed countries sheds light on our own system. For example, Henci Goer in her comprehensive work, *Obstetric Myths versus Research Realities*, paraphrases Dutch researchers' description of their birth economics:

> The Netherlands never fell prey to the economic turf wars of other developed countries that resulted in doctors either driving out midwives or subjugating them under obstetricians. Dutch midwives have maintained full autonomy. They train directly as midwives and are not

ARE YOU A GOOD CANDIDATE FOR A HOME BIRTH?

HOME BIRTH IS FOR WOMEN WHO ARE:

- Healthy
- Eating a sound prenatal diet
- Non-smokers
- Able to envision taking an active role in giving birth, with minimal intervention
- Willing to cope with the pain and hard work of labour (without drugs)
- Living where midwives are available
- Labouring where midwives are available
- Labouring within thirty minutes of a hospital
- Able to cover additional expenses (if their insurance coverage is limited to hospital births)

HOSPITAL BIRTH IS FOR WOMEN WHO HAVE:

- Chronic medical problems (e.g., diabetes, high blood pressure)
- A prenatal problem (e.g., gestational diabetes, preterm labour, preeclampsia, breech, or at least two weeks overdue)
- A desire to birth in a hospital and/or have access to drugs
- Strong fear and/or mistrust of birth as a natural process
- Planned a home birth, but whose labour did not progress normally

required to hold a nursing degree. They provide primary maternity care, while obstetricians are reserved for problematic pregnancies or births. Dutch insurance reimburses only for midwifery care, unless medical problems mandate referral to an obstetrician. *If a woman elects an obstetrician's care, she must pay for it herself* [emphasis added]. Thus, public health policy in the Netherlands has never been shaped by the medical model—the belief that universal hospital confinement is necessary for safety and that the liberal use of interventions is both necessary and harmless. As a result, women may choose home or hospital, and home birth in the Netherlands has remained a viable option, with about one third of women having their babies at home.[2]

IS HOMEBIRTH SAFE?: THE RESEARCH

As the hospital became the unquestioned place to have a baby, medical interventions became the accepted birth rituals. In the last twenty years, most babies in the Western world were born drugged, in an electronic, clinical environment, and separated from their mothers. This turnaround was motivated by a concern for safety, yet paradoxically there is mounting evidence that birth complications *rise* as the utilization of routine technology increases.[4,5]

LEAVING HOME

In 1927, 85 percent of all births in the United States took place at home. Even in the mid-1940's the majority of births still occurred at home (55 percent). Incredibly, by 1973, 91 percent of babies were born in the hospital.[3]

After reviewing available research as to whether moving childbirth to the hospital made birth safer, Henci Goer in her book, *Obstetric Myths versus Research Realities*, reported that "the answer is unequivocally no … Modern techniques and technology still have not succeeded in making hospital birth safer than home birth."[6]

In his article, "The Transition from Home to Hospital Birth in the

United States, 1930–1960" (1977), Neal Devitt reported that "while the techniques of modern hospital obstetrics have saved the lives of many women and infants from genuine pathologies of birth, the literature of obstetrics in the United States from 1930 to 1960 does not show that healthy women with normal pregnancies benefitted from hospital obstetric care … most of the comparative studies of home and hospital birth from the period show that the incidence of birth injuries and obstetric mortality was greater in hospitals, probably due to interference in the normal birth process."[7]

*

Maternal and newborn mortality rates have dropped since the 1930s. There are those who credit the move from home to hospital birth for these improved outcomes. However, Marjorie Tew, a research statistician at Nottingham Medical School, linked the decrease in perinatal mortality with the overall improvement in the health and nutrition of parents, and the availability of antibiotics.

"Since mortality has consistently been higher under obstetric management, extending this to more and more births cannot have been instrumental in reducing the PNMR [perinatal mortality rate]. Statistical analysis of the two trends confirms that increased hospitalization actually kept the PNMR from falling as much as it would inevitably have done in step with the improving health of parents."[8]

*

A significant explosion of misinformation and mistrust in the safety of home birth occurred in 1978 when the American College of Obstetricians and Gynecologists released a widely-published report, "Health Department Data Shows Danger of Home Births." This document stated that "out-of-hospital births pose a two to five times greater risk to a baby's life than hospital birth." The incidence of home birth, which was steadily rising at the time, was undermined by this intellectually sloppy report.

The most glaring fault discrediting the conclusions of this report was the fact that the data on "home births" actually included *all* out-of-hospital births. Outcomes of planned, attended home births involving healthy, full-term, low-risk mothers were lumped together with unattended births that occurred at home or en route to the hospital, and with mothers who may have been high-risk, had not received prenatal care, or were preterm. Unbelievably, the report also included miscarriages in its statistics showing the "risks" of home birth![9]

*

The Farm is a 1,700 acre commune in Summertown, Tennessee, founded in 1971 by Stephen and Ina May Gaskin. The trained and skilled midwives there have professional consulting relationships with physicians, and refer mothers with complications or risk factors to the hospital.

The Duran study (1992) compared 1,700 home births attended by The Farm midwives between 1971 and 1989 to a sample of 14,033 physician-attended births in 1980. The study excluded hospital-mothers with risk factors that would have made them ineligible to birth at The Farm.

The Caesarean rate among mothers who received prenatal care at The Farm was only 1.5 percent compared to 16.5 percent in the doctor-attended group. The transfer-to-hospital rate was 13.5 percent. There was no significant difference between the two groups for perinatal death, bleeding, birth injury, or respiratory distress syndrome. [10]

*

Lewis Mehl, et al, (1977) studied birth outcomes from the medical records of 1,146 elective home births (in the San Francisco area between 1970 and 1975).

The researchers found that among the planned home births in their study, the perinatal mortality rate (foetal and neonatal deaths) was 9.5 per 1000 births, compared to California birth statistics of 1973 showing a perinatal mortality rate of 20.3 per 1000. Mehl, et al, commented, "This is a self-selected, healthy group of women screened for obvious problems and complications occurring during pregnancy, so the data presented here are not directly comparable to state statistics. Still their outcomes are better than average, and the complications rates lower than expected."[11]

In a lecture presented at the annual meeting of The American Foundation for Maternal and Infant Health (1976), Dr. Mehl described other research findings from his comparison of matched, low-risk mothers (1,046 planning home births with 1,046 planning hospital births):

> The hospital-birth women were more likely than the planned home birth mothers to have had the following: five times more likely to have high blood pressure in labour, nine times more likely to have a severe perineal tear, three times more likely to have had postpartum haemorrhage, and three times more likely to have had a Caesarean.

The babies born to the hospital birth women also had a higher complication rate than the babies born to home birth women. In the hospitals, the infants were six times more likely to have had foetal distress before birth, four times more likely to have needed assistance to start breathing, and four times more likely to have developed an infection. There were no birth injuries at home, but thirty infants in the hospital suffered birth injuries.[12]

*

Sullivan and Beeman (1983) studied 1449 clients accepted for prenatal and home birth care with licensed midwives in Arizona between 1978 and 1981. Fourteen percent of the mothers were transferred to the hospital for delivery (complications included lack of progress in labour, preterm labour, meconium staining, foetal distress, or abnormal presentation of the baby, e.g., breech). Of the 1,243 mothers who delivered at home, labour was shorter and the estimated blood loss was less in midwife-assisted home births than normally observed in hospital births. There were three foetal and two neonatal deaths (both from congenital anomalies incompatible with life). The incidence of perinatal mortality among home-birthed babies in this study (4 per thousand) is comparable to low-risk hospital-born babies.[13]

*

Responding to an earlier survey which found that only 8 percent of pregnant women preferred to have their labour at home, Anne Fleissig and Ann Cartwright noted: "Preferences are difficult to study because they are not usually based on experiences of the possible alternatives … One of our studies found that 91 percent of the women who had had their last baby at home said that they would prefer to have their next baby at home, compared with 15 percent of those who had had their baby in hospital. Among the few women who had experienced both a home birth and a hospital birth, 76 percent preferred the home birth."[14]

THE SECOND TIME AROUND

Tom Joles is Albuquerque's local NBC–affiliate evening news co-anchor. I was watching the news when the home birth of his second child, Max, was announced. In response to my note requesting an interview, Tom and his wife, Pat Peterman, graciously invited me to their home. They candidly discussed their decision to have a home birth, the reactions from their friends, and the birth itself.

*

P.E.: How did you come to choose home birth?
PAT: I think the motivation to have a home birth came from my first birth, which took place in a hospital and was everything I didn't want.

I began having contractions early in the week but everyone told me it was false labour. The doctor said if I didn't progress by Friday I would be induced. We weren't bold enough to challenge him. So we went in and let the doctor induce labour and one thing led to another. I had an IV. I wasn't allowed to get out of bed except to go to the bathroom, which drove me crazy.

The external and the internal [monitor] were strapped around me. Every time the baby's heartbeat did anything, everyone came rushing in and panicked!

The doctor broke my water. Then they gave me an epidural because I wasn't relaxed enough, and they started the pitocin [oxytocin drip]. When I was completely dilated, the doctor said I could either wait two hours [until the epidural wore off so I could push], which would cause stress on the baby, or he could use the vacuum extractor and forceps and pull the baby out.

By that time we had pretty much given up and given over, so we allowed them to do that. He used the vacuum extractor and forceps.

I wasn't allowed to touch my baby. I didn't even see our baby for ten minutes. I didn't know what they were doing—they were testing and weighing and doing all these things. I finally had to *ask* to see and to hold our baby.

I came away feeling like I had lost all control of the situation and it plagued me for months. I eventually went to the hospital and talked to the nurses. I went over the record minute by minute to try to find out what happened, why it happened, and understand the decisions we made, so that I could reconcile it. I felt somewhat better when I left, but still felt control had been taken away from me and I still came away feeling I had been cheated.

TOM: We went to the hospital with a game plan and by the time we left it was shredded into about fifty pieces and thrown into the wind and blown all over Albuquerque. We had lost control of the situation.

I don't know if this is the way men think, but I walked away from the hospital thinking, "We have a child in our arms, the child is healthy and that's the most important thing." I was willing to accept what happened in the hospital … *because you have your babies in the hospital.* That's just the way things are.

*

Later, when Pat was pregnant with their second child, the issue of home birth resurfaced. Tom candidly spoke about his decision-making process:

TOM: Having a home birth was initially Pat's idea, and I was *solidly* against it. I looked at the situation and thought, "There's all this technology in the hospital. There are all these highly trained professionals at the hospital. Other people are having babies in the hospital. It only makes sense that we have our child at the hospital."

Then Pat got me thinking and reading about birth. I got to thinking, "It's almost as if you're not having a baby at the hospital—they are waging some kind of war at the hospital." They have all of these sophisticated weapons and trained people over there, and if you know anything about war, when one side has weapons there's a tendency to use them and there's gonna be problems.

I don't think people in hospitals are bad people at all, in fact they have very good intentions. But their instruments sometimes get in the way instead of helping, and their attitudes get in the way too.

*

P.E.: Pat, talk more about your decision to have a home birth.

PAT: I always wanted to birth at home, but for some reason the first time around I was too scared … I was so unsure of myself the first time that I put it in the back of my mind thinking, "Well maybe it's not for me." The second time I got pregnant, the idea came back up in the front of my mind and I started thinking "Well, why not? What's stopping me?"

I began reading and talking to some people who had had home births. After talking to a few midwives, I realized "This wasn't something only *other* people did, it was something we could do … I could do!

*

Tom and Pat consider themselves mainstream, even conventional. Initially their decision to have a home birth surprised a lot of people. Here's what they had to say about the reactions from friends and coworkers:

TOM: What I found really interesting was once I became convinced we should have a home birth, I was into it entirely—but the rest of society wasn't. No one understood us, they thought we were totally bonkers, bananas, wacko … Our decision had made us outsiders and people reacted in a number of ways. Some treated us like we were crazy, others treated us like we were immature, and some acted like we were irresponsible.

PAT: People asked me, "Have you thought about what you're gonna do if something goes wrong?" Of course! That's the first question that comes to mind. They'd say things like, "I know the cord is gonna be wrapped around the child's neck, then what are you gonna do?"

People didn't think about what they were saying. It's a good thing we were sure about what we were doing. We were able to laugh at it as "Boy, there's a lot of ignorance out there," rather than think, "Oh

God, what if the cord is wrapped around the neck?" My thought was, "If the cord is wrapped around our baby's neck, our midwife will flip it off ... no big deal."

TOM: People at work started coming up to me and saying, "I'm really worried about you guys. I'm worried about Pat, I'm worried about the baby, and you—are you sure you can't have the baby in the hospital, would that be too much to ask of you?"

PAT: It's the guilt thing when people come up to you and ask, "Have you really thought about this?" Suddenly you find yourself thinking (but I was able to go past this),"Am I being selfish? Irresponsible? Yes, things occasionally go wrong; am I willing to accept responsibility if something does happen, and live with it the rest of my life?"

TOM: Toward the end I was getting very defensive of our decision: "She's not sick—she's having a baby!" Birth is looked at like a disease ... an emergency. That sums up how people think about birthing.

*

P.E.: What else did you consider before having a home birth?

TOM: There's the guilt and there's also the fear of pain a lot of people talk about. Women have said to me, "When I go in for an appendectomy I certainly get pain killers because it hurts. If I have a baby it's gonna hurt as much if not more, so why not have a pain killer?"

"Many parents and health professionals believe that serious labour complications cause foetal asphyxia and that foetal asphyxia can cause permanent brain damage such as cerebral palsy in the newborn. Those who believe that by identifying peri-natal asphyxia, EFM [external foetal monitoring] can prevent neurologic impairment have unrealistic expectations of this technology. In fact, EFM has not decreased the incidence of cerebral palsy. Over the past 40 years, the rate of cerebral palsy has not changed and remains at about two per 1,000 live births."[15]

– LEAH ALBERS, CNM, DRPH
CHILDBIRTH INSTRUCTOR MAGAZINE

But if you also understand labour's mileposts, you also understand how the hospital can manipulate your thinking. For instance, right before you start pushing, most women are gonna want to bag it, put out a white flag: "I can't take it any more!"

If you can just hold on and view it as a *good* sign—rather than a negative, then you're gonna be able to pull this thing off.

But when you're in a bed in a hospital and they are ready to pounce on you to MAKE YOU FEEL BETTER, to make this "easier", of course you're gonna say, "You're right. I'm really in pain. This is a disgusting experience. Help me out—give me drugs."

*

P.E.: How did you deal with pain during your home birth?

PAT: One book we read said there are some women who can go through the experience and feel no pain because they relax so effectively. Just a few minutes into the experience, once my bag of water broke, I remember saying, "I don't think I can relax, I don't think this relaxation stuff is gonna work!"

TOM: So then we went into the hot tub, and immediately she said, "This is so much better." Being in the hot tub, looking at the stars out there, worked for about 40 minutes. Over time she began to make these noises … and (laughing) I thought to myself, "If the Loch Ness monster were harpooned, that's what it would have sounded like!"

*

When their nurse-midwife determined it was time to push, Pat and Tom went inside to their bedroom.

PAT: Being in our own bedroom, in our house, people could come and go as they wished. It was very relaxed and peaceful. (Tom's parents also attended the birth.)

Afterwards we all sat around and talked, we had champagne and a party. It was a celebration! We did it! It was not a "Whew, I'm glad that's over" kind of experience.

*

P.E.: What did people say after the birth of your baby at home?

TOM: Women have come to me and said, "I've always wanted to have a home birth but I don't think I'm brave enough."

PAT: People have treated me as if I'm heroic, saying "We're so proud of you … We're amazed … It's just miraculous." When people say to me, "You're so brave to have your baby at home," I can only say, "I think you're brave to have your baby in the hospital."

I didn't do anything amazing here, I simply had a baby and I happened to have it at home and that's all there is to it."

Checklist For A Home Birth

LIST OF IMPORTANT PHONE NUMBERS (POSTED BY THE PHONE)

Midwives:

Physician:

Paediatrician:

Preferred Hospital L&D:

Ambulance number:

Your address and home phone number:

☐ Car with fuel & blanket

BIRTH ROOM

☐ 2 sets of sheets and pillow cases
☐ plastic mattress cover or shower curtain
☐ old blanket (for floor delivery)
☐ package of disposable underpads (23″ × 36″)
☐ garbage bucket and plastic bags
☐ 3 bath towels
☐ 6–8 washcloths

- [ ] inflatable bath pillow or doughnut
- [ ] camera and film
- [ ] tape recorder (to record first cry)

FOR MOTHER

- [ ] 3–4 litres juice or sports drinks
- [ ] ice
- [ ] 2 knee-length T-shirts or gowns
- [ ] incense or aromatherapy oils
- [ ] overnight and regular sanitary pads
- [ ] Mother's Milk tea
- [ ] 2–3 bags of Sitz Bath Herbs
- [ ] sitz bath (optional, inexpensive)
- [ ] Ibuprofen or paracetamol (for afterpains)
- [ ] heating pad

FOOD FOR BIRTH COMPANIONS
& POSTPARTUM MEAL

- [ ] high protein/fruit/chocolate snacks
- [ ] your postpartum meal

FOR BABY

Have ready at the bedside:
- [ ] 6 receiving blankets
- [ ] 1 nappy (disposable preferable)
- [ ] 1 undershirt
- [ ] 1 sleeper or kimono
- [ ] 1 pair socks
- [ ] 1 cotton knit cap or bonnet
- [ ] thermometer

FOR CORD CARE:

- [ ] Q-tips
- [ ] hydrogen peroxide or alcohol
- [ ] rosemary, arrowroot or goldenseal

WHAT MODERN HOME BIRTH MIDWIVES BRING

Midwives usually bring along another experienced midwife and/or an obstetric nurse to assist in case another pair of hands is needed. In case you're curious, here's a list of what you'd find in a midwife's home-birth bag:

- Your chart, including your prenatal records and lab work
- Foetascope and/or doppler
- Blood pressure cuff and stethoscope
- Thermometer
- Sterile gloves, water-soluble jelly and betadine solution
- Sterile birth pack (which includes haemostats, scissors, cord clamp or tie, 4x4 gauze)
- Amnihook—to break your water if necessary
- Bulb and DeLee suction for the baby
- Syntocin (oxytocin) and Methergine, drugs to stimulate uterine contractions after the placenta is delivered in order to control heavy bleeding (Note: syntocin inductions in labour are never done at home)
- IV bags, tubing and catheters
- Oxygen
- Ambu bag—in case a baby needs a little help getting breathing started
- Sterile suture material, drapes, scissors, needle holder and Lignocaine or Lidocaine (to numb a tear or episiotomy that needs to be repaired)
- Sterile catheters—should you need help emptying your bladder
- Herbs, oils, aromatherapy
- Vitamin K for the baby
- A baby scale and measuring tape to get your baby's birth weight and length

Note: Midwives notify the Department of Health of the child's birth, but parents must register the birth at their local Register Office.

*

BIRTHING WHERE YOU'LL BE "AT HOME"

Make a whole-hearted effort to choose the environment which resonates with your beliefs. For example, one mother told me she considered birthing in a small community hospital with an excellent reputation for flexibility and personal attention. While taking the tour of the birth centre, she realized she "would feel much safer in a busy hospital with lots of people around, in case there was an emergency."

Fortunately, this mother was in touch with her deep-seated fears. Attempting to birth in a low-key birth centre or at home probably would have generated enough anxiety to stop labour or create a problem that might have brought her into the hospital anyway. In this situation, choosing a busy, high-tech hospital environment probably improved her chances of birthing normally.

Home birth is not for everyone. Goer concludes:

> Ultimately the issue of the safety of home birth cannot be settled by research … It comes down to a matter of individual choice. The real question about safety is not, "Do you want a pleasant birth at home or a safe birth in the hospital?" It is, "Do you want to give birth at home and run the minuscule risk of an emergency that might (but not necessarily would) be handled better in the hospital, or do you want to give birth in the hospital and run the considerably increased risk of infection, the certainty of additional stress, and the near certainty of having unnecessary (and potentially risky) interventions?"[16]

Like all important decisions in our lives, *choosing* where we birth involves gathering and sorting through information, exploring our values and priorities, and, finally, taking responsibility for our choices.

*

If you decide you want to give birth at home, then your next task is to choose a skilled birth attendant. This is an important decision not unlike choosing other professionals (e.g., a lawyer, mechanic, or surgeon) whose experience and expertise you will want to trust. In any profession there's a wide range of competence, so get references and do careful interviewing before selecting your birth attendant (regardless of where you plan to birth).

Being Powerful in Birth

Chapter 20

Even Paper Tigers Can Bite

Imagine yourself labouring in the jungle. Suppose you saw, or even thought you saw, a hungry tiger lurking in the nearby shadows. What do you think would happen to your labour?

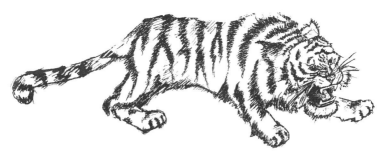

You may think you have a choice in this situation, but your body has already made the decision Believing there's a tiger in your birth space instantly would stimulate a healthy "fight or flight" reaction. Labour contractions would slow down or stop and not resume until you felt safe.

No mother can give birth if she feels unsafe or senses danger. Fear activates the nervous system to produce adrenalin, which fuels the "fight or flight" response. This increases heart and respiratory rates and shunts blood away from internal organs (including the uterus) to the large muscles. Increased levels of adrenalin also neutralize the effect of oxytocin (the hormone responsible for stimulating uterine contractions).

Therefore, if your personal imagery triggers excessive fear during pregnancy, you may never go into labour. If you do enter labour, your contractions may not be powerful enough to get the baby out. Conversely, when your image of birth is one of safety and strength, your nervous system will respond accordingly, producing a state of relaxation, a normal heart and respiratory rate, and strong, effective contractions.

The autonomic nervous system is not able to discriminate between real or imagined "tigers". It simply responds to imagery. That's why it's important to bring your images, beliefs and fears to *conscious* awareness, where you can tame, eliminate, or even harness them.

DON'T BE YOUR OWN "TIGER"

We've all had the experience of being frightened or worried by one of our own fantasies. You've probably already scared yourself at least once with your imagination during this pregnancy (perhaps while reading about complications or waiting for the results of a prenatal test). In labour's trance, you will be even more vulnerable to being scared by your unresolved fears and by the worries of others. If you are scaring yourself, just ask:

- What am I *telling* myself?
- Is this actually *happening*, or am I fantasizing it?

Whenever you scare yourself it means you've left your moment-to-moment awareness. Realize the fantasy is in your head and bring yourself back to the moment by practising non-focused awareness.

GEORGIA'S STORY:

Georgia, a neonatal ICU nurse, was planning to give birth in the same hospital where she worked. While tracking her tigers, she realized she was dreading labour-visits from her many well-meaning colleagues. Georgia was concerned about privacy, performance anxiety and how she'd be affected by co-workers' concerns about her baby's well-being.

In her eighth month, Georgia finally looked her tigers in the eye. Then she graciously explained her wishes to her colleagues and invited them to visit the day after her baby was born. In addition, she asked her husband to make a big, colourful sign to hang on her labour door that stated: MOTHER AT WORK! Thanks for Your Support, But NO Visitors!

Georgia expressed a sense of relief and relaxation after taming this tiger.

TRY THIS: TRACKING YOUR TIGERS

There's a difference between fleeting anxieties and dangerous tigers. Dangerous tigers trigger recurrent tight feelings in your gut, nightmares and constant worry. They can be real or imagined (e.g., a hostile birth attendant, or the *worry* you'll have to deal with one).

If either of these kind of tigers is lurking, take action. Pretending it's not there, or ignoring it hoping it will go away, is a sign that you think it's bigger and stronger than you are. You may be able to keep it at bay in pregnancy, but during the vulnerability of labour it will be on the prowl. (If in the throes of labour an unexpected tiger shows up, don't freeze. You or your birth companion can cage that tiger, too). Here's how to track your tigers:

1. Write down all the things you hope won't happen.
2. Look your tigers in the eye. (Let your imagination flow into your fear.)
3. Ask yourself: What do I need to do to tame or escape each tiger? (i.e., what will make my birth place safe?).
4. DO IT! (Even if you are afraid.) Get help if you need it.

Chapter 21

Labour Means Hard Work

One day I asked Suzanne Stalls, a midwife in Albuquerque, how she prepares women for labour. Seasoned by attending hundreds of women in birth, both at home and in the hospital, Suzanne has developed a sixth sense about labour. She said she tries to instill confidence in her mothers by telling them:

> There are three things that are givens about labour: It's hard work, it hurts a lot, and you can do it. That's the bottom line. All the rest you learn about is icing on the cake.

This icing can come in different flavors. Couples who've experienced or fear sterile, impersonal, stainless steel delivery rooms may react by creating a warm, romantic fantasy of birth-by-candlelight. Suzanne speaks candidly about this phenomenon:

> When I arrive at a labouring couple's home and find candles burning, soft music playing and the mother wearing a flowing, white lace nightgown, I know we're in trouble. I think to myself, "Uh-oh, this is going to take a long time." I know I can either get out my knitting and settle in, or snuff the candles, turn off the music, and throw her an old T-shirt. In other words, tell her to get down to work.

I give this handout (Figure 21.1) to parents in my childbirth classes to take with them in labour as a visual reminder of things that might be helpful. I used drawings instead of words to speak to their "right" brain. Here are some things to think about:

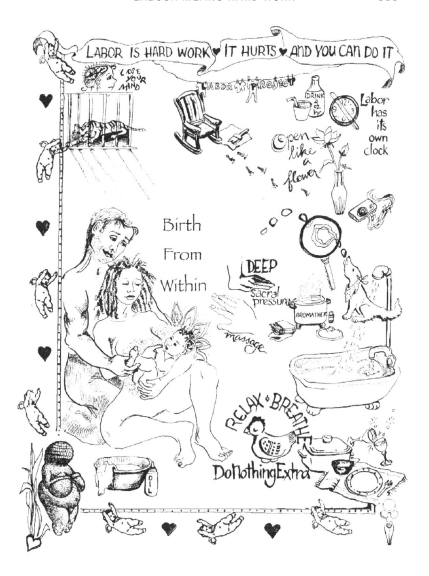

FIGURE 21.1 Birthing From Within © 1997. Intended for private use by parents and may not be reproduced for publication or educational purposes without permission.

LABOUR HAS ITS OWN CLOCK

A watched kettle never boils …
and a timed uterus never contracts.

Actually, a watched kettle only seems like it never boils because of the effect that watching has on our perception of time. A uterus, however, doesn't just *seem* to slow down when our attention is focused on it: its functioning actually *is* affected by being "watched."

A slowly unfolding labour may produce anxiety in those around you. Watching contraction after contraction is boring, and there may be concern about your ability to cope with prolonged discomfort. Those attending may want to do something to speed labour up, or rescue you from your "misery."

For the first time in history, labour patterns are being timed, assessed and charted. Sometimes this information is helpful to midwives and doctors. Legitimate issues concerning time should be managed by your birth attendants (it's *their* job!). But when mothers and fathers become preoccupied with timing every contraction, it's a different story.

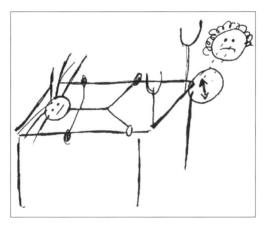

FIGURE 21.2 "The MD's looking at the doctor s clock to make sure they're not being kept too long. Metal, everything is metal, not soft. Even her hair, theres no softness about her. I accidentally did the hair that way … she's scared out of her wits."

AMY

When you, or your contraction pattern, are watched too closely, you become self-conscious. Amy said of her 20-hour labour, (Figure 21.2,) "I was worried after about 10 hours that I was moving too slowly, that I was running out of time on the doctor's clock."

This time-orientation forces labouring women to remain intellectually focused: to think about how long they have suffered; how much longer they must suffer; and how fast or slow labour is progressing. They worry whether their labour will be fast enough to "beat the doctor's clock." Women believe, not without reason, that if they don't labour fast enough, various interventions, including a Caesarean, may be implemented.

So, forget everything you have learned about stages or patterns of labour. Labour is simply a series of contractions that ease open the mouth of your womb and push out your baby. Primitive women, even your grandmothers, didn't need to know about stages of labour, and neither do you. You should forget about keeping track of time.

When you allow yourself to become immersed in labour, it is neither boring nor interesting, because the very nature of labour dissolves ordinary boundaries of time and space. You and labour become one. Timing your labour requires remaining conscious-of-self rather than *being-in-labour*.

Once your uterus knows it's not being watched and timed, its performance anxiety will be relieved.

LABOUR PROJECT

The burst of energy that accompanies the onset of labour allows for last minute "nesting." Use this opportunity to take care of any unfinished business before settling into your birth place and the state-of-mindlessness sometimes referred to as "Labourland."

In America, the image of women in labour lying down in a narrow bed, waiting, and watching the monitor has become part of our idea of birth. Yet, some women don't accept the role of passive-patient. I remember the impact on me of Katie's labour story as told by Penny Armstrong in her book, *A Midwife's Story*.

My first delivery was in an Amish cottage, fenced in with an honest-to-goodness white picket fence. I turned into the drive just as Enos, the father, was tucking his two-year-old onto the seat of an open buggy … [he] waved, grinned, and said he'd be right back …

Thinking I would find Katie stretched out in her bed, I turned to go up the steps to the back porch. Just then she popped out the back door. She had a paintbrush in her hand.

"Oh," she said, "hi. Oh, my goodness, I'm not quite ready. I was putting the final coat of lacquer on this rocking chair when I started to have stronger contractions. I just wanted so much for it to be done, so I could rock the baby in it." …

She'd cleaned the brush and now she laid it down on some neatly folded newspapers spread out on a corner of the porch. Not only did the rocker look freshly lacquered, but it appeared that the porch floor had been scrubbed and waxed not long ago. She stopped talking for a moment when she stood up, put her hands on her hips, and stretched out her back.

"Is that a contraction?" I asked.

"Yes it is."

"Is it pretty strong?"

"Yes, I believe it is, and I haven't put that plastic thing on the bed yet."

We walked through an immaculate kitchen and a spotless living room. She'd gotten her husband off to work, gotten her toddler up, washed, fed, and dressed, cleaned up the breakfast dishes, straightened up the living room, and painted a rocking chair. I think it was about 8:30 in the morning. I had my small bag in my hand.

"Before we make the bed, let's see how dilated you are." I was thinking that this woman couldn't be too far along since she was running around like she was getting ready for her first date.

Wrong. Nine centimeters.

"Where's that plastic sheet?" I said. "Looks to me like you're about to have a baby."

She chattered her way off to the linen closet and back. "Oh, I'm so excited," she said. "I can hardly wait. Every night when I go to bed, I say to Enos, 'Maybe tonight I'll have the baby. Maybe by tomorrow it will be lying right there between us. …

She stopped again for another contraction, and as soon as it passed she went back to spreading out the plastic sheet over the mattress cover …

We finished making up the bed, then she thought maybe she'd change from her dress into a gown. Next thing I knew, she'd hopped onto the bed. Her face was flushed and she was ready to push …

Enos arrived just as she was getting serious about pushing. He went to Katie's side and grabbed her hand.

The three of us attended quietly. A couple of times Katie said it hurt and she called her husband's name, and he got closer to her and held her so she could push more easily. The baby, a boy, popped out … l put him on the bed at Katie's side, and she curled herself around him.

"Oh," she said, "look at him … Look at our new baby … Oh, my, look how beautiful he is. Just look. Oh, Enos, I love him already.'"

For Katie, giving birth was part of living, and she didn't stop living to give birth. Rather than keeping track of the stages of labour, she was busy doing things which strengthened her bond to her baby.

Katie's story inspired me to plan a labour project of my own. Luc was due a week before Christmas, and we had just cut and decorated a small tree. I left tinseling of the tree for my labour project.

A good labour project involves physical movement, contact with your normal daily life, and mental engagement in a way that blocks obsessive focusing on your labour process. Here are a few ideas for labour projects:

- Bringing photo album up to date
- Sewing something for the baby
- Cutting quilt pieces
- Gardening (sink your fingers into the earth)
- Baking a birthday cake, cookies or favorite casserole to eat after the baby's born
- Washing and folding baby clothes
- Writing letters or holiday cards
- Cleaning your cupboards

ON YOUR OWN TWO FEET

Well-intentioned, but excessive, support in early labour (as when a birth companion hovers solicitously) can make you feel helpless, weak, and dependent.

When you are in early labour, contractions are mild, and you won't have entered Labourland yet—so you don't need "support." You're not helpless; you are strong and about to have a baby. Nothing needs to be done for you, yet.

It is better for both you and your birth companion to be involved in a labour project, either together or on your own. Remember, early (mild) labour is preparing the cervix for active or hard labour, and this phase can take hours.

WHEN TO GO TO THE HOSPITAL

Often couples are told to go to the hospital when contractions are five minutes apart for an hour. Experienced birth attendants, who know that it is easier to labour at home, sometimes will encourage couples to stay home until labour has progressed further.

Sometimes with a first baby, it can take several hours to a day of regular, mild contractions to ripen and thin the cervix *before* labour is considered "active" or hard. So unless you have a special condition or for personal reasons prefer to be in the hospital in early labour, stay home and get busy with your labour project.

When you can no longer focus on your labour project or you feel spacey or restless between contractions, it usually means you are moving along and it's time to go. Midwives at University Hospital in Albuquerque tell their mums to bake chocolate chip cookies in early labour— "when the cookies start burning [because you're entering Labourland], it's time to come in."

EATING, DRINKING, AND STAYING STRONG

There was a period in American obstetrics when women were routinely advised not to eat or drink anything (except ice chips) after labour began. This was to prevent vomiting under general anaesthesia during the rare event of an emergency Caesarean.

The reality is that labouring women, like athletes, become dehydrated. Dehydration and starvation can lead to dysfunctional labour. Hospitals recognize this, so when a woman is dehydrated or is exhausted from low blood sugar, they start an IV. The mother's freedom of movement is thereby restricted, however, making it harder for her to do the moving around she senses will help her.

To avoid dehydration in labour, drink at least a quarter of a pint per hour: choose drinks that replace sugar or electrolytes—cold juice, tea with honey, miso soup, sports drinks, popsicles or iced-juice chips. (Orange juice tends to make women vomit.)

It's important to eat something every two or three hours in early labour, since you don't know how long it will last. This way you won't be in a fasting state when the hard work of active labour begins! You'll probably want to eat something light, e.g., fruit, yoghurt, cereal, soft-boiled egg and toast. You will lose your appetite when active labour begins.

The worst that can happen from eating in labour is throwing up. That probably isn't part of your birth fantasy, but in the depths of Labourland you won't really care. But if you haven't eaten anything, the penalty of exhaustion and starvation can reduce your endurance in labour.

MUSIC

As in aerobics classes, where music is part of the driving energy to get the workout done, the right music may help you move with the rhythm of labour.

If you are birthing in a hospital, music can bring familiarity to a strange room. Wearing headphones can shut out distracting hospital noises.

STOP THINKING

It's much easier to manage labour's intensity if you're not intellectualizing about what's happening or obsessing about what to do.

Other mammals birth instinctively simply because there is no thinking about the right way to do it or what stage they are in. Nature has its own ways of anaesthetizing a human's brilliant intellectual development to allow birth to happen naturally. Labour works better when you're out of your mind.

RELAX, BREATHE, FEEL THE EARTH; DO NOTHING EXTRA

In Zen, there is a teaching: "Do nothing extra." Students are taught to do what needs to be done, with their whole body-mind, but without extra gestures, chatter, or effort; nothing extra. This practice is described beautifully in *The Healing Art of Tai Chi* by Martin Lee, et al:

> What does a hen have to do to ensure the birth of her chicks? Just four things: relax, breathe, feel the earth beneath her, and then do nothing extra. These actions prevent stress that could adversely affect her unhatched eggs. If the hen feels stress, she may not be able to stay warm, and then her eggs may not hatch. If the hen does something extra, there will not be any chicks. For example, during the hatching process, the hen often gets up and turns the eggs over. Doing nothing extra means she does nothing unnecessary. She does not jump up and down on the eggs, poke holes to see if they are ready to hatch, or take 10-minute breaks. She simply instinctively turns them over.
>
> … Chickens, like most creatures in nature, learn how to live without any coaching. They know how to relax, breathe, feel the ground, and do nothing extra …
>
> [At first you may find] doing nothing extra the most difficult of these four elements. It simply means carry out each task as naturally and instinctively as you can, allowing nature to meet you halfway. The less you do the more nature will do for you.[2]

GETTING DOWN AND DIRTY

Soldiers are trained to give everything in battle. They expect to return from war grimy, sweaty, dishevelled, and sometimes even bloody; it's their badge of honour. Likewise, a gutsy football or baseball player who ends the game wearing a uniform caked with mud is perceived as having given his all. Some cultures (but not ours) honour women in the same way when they return from battling in the trenches of labour.

"Most Western women have never been physically tested until we go through labor and birth ... haven't gone eighteen or twenty-four hours without food or sleep ... allowed ourselves to go a day or two ... without a bath or shower, without brushing our teeth and doing our hair and makeup. Even fewer of us would allow anyone else to see, smell, or touch us, unwashed, sweat-soaked, naked, oozing mucus, blood, and feces from our nether regions. When faced with the forces of labor, we can't hide the fear, the anxiety, the responses to pain ... All the inhibitions and trappings of our social selves are peeled away as our bodies thrust and heave, vomit and grunt, cry and leak. The animal is there for everyone to see."[3]

SUSAN DIAMOND, R.N.
HARD LABOR

Wouldn't it be great if childbirth teachers and health professionals instilled that same tough mindset in mothers and fathers? Rather than promoting the reassuring, but unlikely, illusion of being comfortable and relaxed in labour, teachers should help mothers and fathers muster the courage and determination to get through it. That's why Birthing From Within works at helping couples prepare to face the rigours of "battling with nature," without fleeing the battle field when the going gets tough. Here's how we do it:

First, we help mothers experience themselves as part of a larger whole, a link in the chain of mothers throughout time. We do this using exercises described in Chapter 4.

Second, we explain that to give birth with power, without drugs, means having to go to the edge, and beyond.

Third, we point out that the hospital "battle field," in striving to be sterile and clean, inadvertently sends a confusing message to women giving birth. Birth-warriors don't stay clean, together, made-up, and poised (see above).

Finally, mothers must make a heart-felt commitment: Not to birth normally, but to **give it their all, moment-by-moment**. Once they've *done* that, to then be okay with whatever happens.

As a Birth-Warrior
What do you look like?
What sounds do you make?
What's your battle cry?
How do you show your fearless, fierce nature?
Find the place within yourself where this courage lies.

Chapter 22

Out of Control: How To "Lose It" In Labour

Most women start my classes with the idea (or hope) that I will help them reach their goal of being calm, confident, and controlled in labour. Unfortunately, many professionals feed into these unrealistic expectations (both prenatally and during labour itself). Because I know the difficulties created for mothers by this ideal image, I don't promise (or endorse) those results.

Imagine being in line for your first trip on the Mega-Roller Coaster. All around you terrifying tales are being told about the ride. At the same time, videos are being shown of others riding the roller coaster looking calm and composed.

Instead of feeling normal excitement and anxiety as your adventure nears, you start to become pre-occupied with doing it *right*. You may even begin worrying whether you've got "the right stuff," and how your partner in the next seat will react if he thinks you haven't measured up!

HOW COULD THERE BE JUST ONE RIGHT WAY TO GIVE BIRTH WHEN THERE ARE BILLIONS OF WOMEN IN THIS WORLD?

Usually I hear a collective sigh of relief when I tell the parents in my childbirth classes how for some mothers, moaning … groaning … wailing … rocking … white-knuckling … and "losing control" … may actually be their *key* to getting their baby out, naturally.

What each woman needs to do in labour reflects her individuality. In addition, a mother may need to be different in one labour than she might in a subsequent one. "Natural labour" means doing what comes naturally, for *you*.

A woman who is quiet in many situations, may be quiet during childbirth. On the other hand, a verbally and physically effusive woman is likely to be the same way in labour. For *that* woman to attempt to stifle her self-expression because she (or someone else) thinks she should, would be *unnatural*, and unproductive.

The goal of maintaining control and relaxation has been a powerful force in promoting the use of drugs in labour. If you're giving birth in a hospital, you may run into professionals who still consider drugs and anaesthesia to be their only ways of helping you when you are in pain. So that's what they'll offer.

Inexperienced couples in my classes can't appreciate how powerful the temptation is to accept offers of relief in a painfully vulnerable moment. I remember a mother in one of my childbirth classes who was totally committed to labouring without drugs. She did not believe me when I warned that repeated offers of pain relief wear down a mother's resolve. Later, after giving birth, she told me what had happened:

POWER FROM SURRENDER

"I was so in my head with my first birth, trying to think my way out of this painful dilemma. I squirmed and tried to push away the pain. The pain only intensified. Although I was committed to a natural childbirth, after twenty-four hours of labour I was ready to just cut the baby out. But I knew I really didn't want that.

My midwife in her wisdom sent over a good friend [Mary] who was very jolly and round. Her babies practically fell out of her. Mary positioned herself in bed next to me and said, 'It's just like surfing. Let's ride these contractions.' She taught me how to let go and surf with the force of nature. And then it became bliss.

It occurred to me a lot of [my] pain was caused by resistance to surrender. I was fighting it, trying to get away from the pain. I was judgmental of myself, wondering why I couldn't do it 'right.'

Mary was not in her head. She was completely jolly and happy, and she brought joy into the room. She took me out of my head and into my body."[1]

– A PARTICIPANT'S STORY TOLD IN A SATSANG
WITH GANGAJI FROM THE AUDIOTAPE,
THE FREEDOM OF NO ESCAPE

I was doing fine—I thought. It hurt but I was handling it. When I got into active labour, I began to show my pain more. My nurse was nice enough. She came in to check the monitor every 15 to 20 minutes or so. And every time she came in, she asked, "Ready for your epidural now?"

She never encouraged me or told me I was doing fine … so I guess I started losing confidence and thought maybe I wasn't doing okay. No one told me how much further I had to go, or how close I was …

Finally, after I was worn down and discouraged enough, I said "yes" to the epidural. You know what bothers me most? It's how happy those two nurses seemed about me finally agreeing to the epidural. They kept telling me that now I was doing the right thing.

It isn't just pain or well-intentioned offers of relief that steer women into using drugs they had wanted to do without. It's also their fear of "losing it" in labour, and others' judgements about that, that pushes them to say "yes" to drugs.

How can you and your partner avoid this common scenario? Here's what you can do:

1. Be realistic about your vulnerability in labour. Anticipate that the physiological and psychological state of Labourland will make you highly susceptible to offers of relief.

GANGAJI RESPONDS

"She took you into surrender. She pointed the way for you to surrender. I'm sure she's had clients who've resisted throughout the whole time.

There's some kind of feeling which calls forth resistance and the fear of dissolution. There is the thought 'I will collapse. I will cease to be.' You as you have known yourself does dissolve. Who you think you are dissolves, because who you think you are is built on 'I'm doing well, I'm doing bad.'"

– GANGAJI

2. Recognize the value of privacy during labour.
3. Choose birth companions who believe you can do it, don't see drugs as an inevitable part of labour, and have the tact and assertiveness to communicate with hospital personnel as necessary.
4. Recognize that even among skilled and compassionate medical professionals, there are two basic philosophies. First, there are those who believe you can cope with pain without drugs, who know how to support you through the pain, but who also have the wisdom and experience to recognize labours where drugs may be the best idea. Then there are professionals who consider it unnecessary or foolish to endure any pain that drugs can do away with.

   If your goals *match* the beliefs of the professional on call, or assigned to you, you don't have a problem. However, if a major philosophical discrepancy becomes apparent, here's what needs to be done:

   Your partner (or birth companion) should go to whomever is in charge, explain the kind of support you are looking for, and graciously request that someone different be assigned to work with you. You'll be happier, and the professional originally assigned to you probably will be too.
5. Practise the mindful pain-coping techniques described in Chapter 38.

WHAT IS IT MOST WOMEN ARE AFRAID OF "LOSING?"

I've learned how important it is to ask women the following questions (I never assume I know what "losing it" means to *them*):

- What does "losing it" in labour mean to you?
- What is it you fear about "losing it" in labour?
- How much of your concern is about what you would think about yourself, versus what other people would think about you if you "lost it?"
- If you completely "lost it" in labour, what would you be doing?
- How might "losing it" in labour be *helpful* to you?

Most of us are afraid to give up the image of who we think we are, or are supposed to be. So, when facing the unknown of birth, especially while being bombarded by stories of other women's "successes" or "failures," we hold on even tighter to our ideal image. The desire to maintain that persona often drives the search for magic techniques and perfect birth settings.

Give it up. Expect/accept that you probably will lose something (confidence, "control") at some point during labour. If you feel like you're losing control, accept it, even embrace it. You may be surprised to find that the moment will pass. In fact, fighting the moment feeds and prolongs your sense of desperation.

In Zen there is a saying, "Fall down seven times, get up eight times." This teaching models the tremendous determination and concentration you will need to give birth your way.

Chapter 23

These Bones Were Made for Birthin'

One spring, a group of New Mexico midwives hosted a tea for Ina May Gaskin, author of the landmark book, *Spiritual Midwifery.* I asked what she tells expectant mothers who've had a Caesarean birth for "small bones."

"Let's see," she said thoughtfully. "I have helped a few women who have done beautifully. What I tell women is that they will get big, bigger than the baby. And it works.

"Even doctors allow that the uterus does and will expand sufficiently and naturally in pregnancy. They don't doubt that the uterus can grow and contain a large baby, even twins. But then in labour the beliefs change. Suddenly the cervix can't dilate enough, the bony diameter (of the pelvis) is not big enough."

Ina May explained how (male) doctors could have limited women's consciousness for so long. "You see," she said, "men's consciousness is limited. They can only get so big, and no bigger! But women are not limited. Mothers get bigger than the baby. Not just 10 centimetres, but bigger than the baby."

Ina May went on to explain that "because of men's biological unfamiliarity with birth, men cannot understand the *mystery* of birth (although they have tried to understand through scientific study of birth). But for women who are in touch with their bodies, being pregnant and giving birth is not a 'mystery.' They know what is happening inside them and they can give birth."

YOUR PELVIS AND PELVIMETRY

Your bony pelvis contains and protects your uterus, ovaries, bladder, intestines, and rectum. Your baby will pass through the spacious opening in your pelvis during birth.

During a vaginal exam, midwives and doctors can only *estimate* the diameters of your pelvic bones. This exam is called pelvimetry, and may be helpful in finding gross abnormalities that could interfere with birth. Remember, pelvimetry provides only an estimate; there is a lot of possibility for error.

FIGURE 23.1 (a) Before labour, your baby's skull bones are loosely connected by membranes with spaces between the bones.

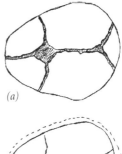

(a)

(b) As your baby's head moves through your pelvis the skull bones move closer together and may even override each other (moulding). This natural adaptation does not hurt your baby's brain because compression in one direction is accompanied by expansion in another.

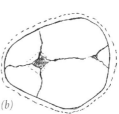

(b)

Just as your breasts and uterus undergo tremendous structural changes as pregnancy progresses, so does your pelvis. By the latter half of pregnancy, hormones will have softened the cartilage and lengthened the tendons and ligaments that hold the pelvic bones together, effectively expanding the opening in your pelvis. You will know this has occurred when you feel your symphysis pubis and hip bones riding up and down when you walk (or waddle).

FIGURE 23.2

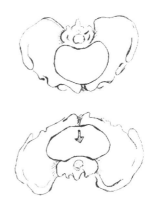

If you are examined in the first half of pregnancy these changes will not have occurred yet. So, if you are told you are "too small" during that first visit, don't worry. Don't starve your hungry, growing baby just because you are told you can only birth a six pound baby. Nobody (not even an ultrasound) can accurately predict what size baby you will have or will be able to deliver. Restricting protein and calories in a misguided effort to grow a smaller baby could result in permanent neurological damage.

True cases of significant pelvic abnormality are rare. Even if someone suspects that to be the case, it's just about impossible to determine whether or not your baby will "fit" before labour. Your pelvic bones are not rigid and immobile during labour; there is continuous, harmonious motion between them and your baby's head.

In addition, your baby's still-malleable skull bones "mould" (overlap) during birth, thus reducing the circumference of its head as it's being born. After birth, the skull bones slide back into their normal position so that within hours, your baby's head is round again (Figure 23.1).

GET UP!

Lying on your back collapses your pelvis, distorting its natural opening, and decreases the diameter by as much as an inch (Figure 23.2). Being upright not only avoids that problem, but allows gravity to work for you. Standing, sitting on the edge of a bed or chair, or being on hands and knees often opens the pelvis just right.

In their wonderful book, *Women Giving Birth,* Astrid Limburg and Beatrijs Smulders describe and illustrate the changes in pelvic diameter in the squatting, semi-sitting and lying flat positions:

> Squatting puts traction on the otherwise relaxed symphysis and increases the pubic arch, the space under the pubic bones, which brings about the necessary rotation of the head in the birth canal. The sacroiliac joint gives the sacrum flexibility. When the trunk bends forward, as it does in the squatting position, the sacrum turns on its axis and opens up the pelvis from behind, increasing the width of the pelvic outlet (Figure 23.3).

FIGURE 23.3

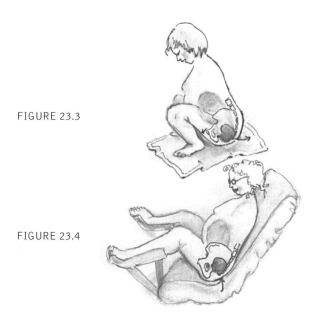

FIGURE 23.4

The semi-sitting position (Figure 23.4), decreases the diameter by: 1) flattening the pelvis from the pressure exerted from the bed; 2) immobilizing the usually mobile coccyx, forcing it into the pelvic cavity; and 3) not exerting tension on the pubic symphisis, thus preventing the widening of the pubic arch.

Although lying flat on your back works against gravity, may decrease the oxygen supply to the baby and increase labour pain, it is better than the semi-sitting position. On your back, at least, the coccyx is unobstructed and the upper part of the body is bent in a way that increases the size of the pelvic opening.[1]

CPD: NOT AN ABSOLUTE DIAGNOSIS

CPD stands for Cephalo Pelvic Disproportion. It refers to a condition where the baby, especially its head, is too large to fit through the mother's bony pelvis.

CPD is the common explanation given to many mothers whose labours fail to progress and end in birth by Caesarean. But this does not mean that the next baby won't fit. A woman who has given birth by Caesarean for CPD often goes on to deliver a *larger* infant normally!

Studies examining the likelihood of VBAC after a previous Caesarean birth for CPD or failure to progress in labour, report an average success rate of 67 percent (with a range from 50 to 80 percent).[2,3,4]

Some doctors and midwives think that CPD is often incorrectly diagnosed, when other causes actually arrested labour progress (such as contractions that weren't strong enough, inactivity, lying down during labour, or not having allowed enough time for the mother's cervix to dilate before making the diagnosis).

In a future labour, if these problems do not recur, or are corrected, a normal birth is possible, even likely. For most women, vaginal birth after a previous Caesarean birth is safe, and in fact, safer than an elective or routine repeat Caesarean. Talk this over with your doctor or midwife.

Chapter 24

Stand and Deliver

Pushing your baby out is a fiercely primitive experience, and hard physical work. However, it is simple in that the urge to push is a reflex that usually arises spontaneously when the time is right. Believe it or not, you already know how to push your baby into the world. You do not need to "learn" how to push your baby out any more than you had to learn other reflexes such as coughing, blinking or sneezing.

In fact, you know better than anyone how, when and where to push your baby out. How could anyone know better than you? You have cradled your baby in your womb and carried him under your heart for months; only you can feel his head moving through your pelvis, and feel your pelvis moving with each contraction. Only you can feel how a shift in your position, as little as an inch in one direction or the other, enhances the strength and harmony of each push.

From childhood, women in previous centuries, as well as those in non-Western cultures, have had the advantage of witnessing women giving birth naturally. Long before their hour to birth arrived, they unconsciously had absorbed an underlying confidence in their bodies' ability to labour and deliver. It makes sense to learn a few helpful guidelines and role-play how to follow them, since most of us haven't witnessed birth.

NOT ALL PUSHING IS EQUAL

There are two approaches to pushing out your baby. One is the forceful approach, and the other is natural or exhale pushing.

FORCEFUL PUSHING

In 1861 a doctor wrote a paper suggesting that the time a mother pushes in labour should never exceed two hours.[1] Unfortunately, this idea (in the absence of sound research), was perpetuated for over a century. The erroneous belief that pushing in childbirth is dangerous to the baby caused physicians to institute practices that have proven more harmful to mothers and babies than natural pushing! One practice is the frequent use of forceps or vacuum extractors. Another is having the mother push before she has the urge or is fully dilated (which can result in either a swollen cervix, and therefore a longer labour, or a torn cervix).

Probably the convention most commonly practiced is forceful (Valsalva manoeuvre) pushing. No mother naturally pushes this way; she has to be taught or persuaded to do this. Here's how it goes:

A mother is often instructed to lie on her back or get into a semi-sitting position. Sometimes stirrups or footrests are used.

When the contraction begins, the nurse tells the mother to take two slow breaths, then hold the third breath and begin pushing to the count of ten. With the vigour of a cheerleader, the nurse shouts at the mother, "P-U-S-H! P-U-S-H! One. Two. Three. Four. Don't waste the contraction! (How can you "waste a contraction?" There are always plenty more.) Six. Seven. Eight. Nine. Ten ... Okay take another breath, Quick, P-U-S-H!! ... One. Two. Three ..."

The mother gains approval according to the degree her face and neck veins become red and distended with blood as she pushes. Sometimes as a result of the forceful pushing, capillaries burst, appearing as little purple spots called petechia, on her face and chest. Her eyes literally appear to bulge out of their sockets. Those caring for her feel confident that the results of this vigourous pushing will be beneficial to both her and her baby.

CONNECTING WITH OTHER WOMEN

Bats usually give birth hanging *upright*, i.e., head up, feet down. But, on one occasion, Boston University biologist Thomas Kunz witnessed an inexperienced fruit bat labouring unsuccessfully while hanging upside-down. A female bat "midwife" flew over to her, and for three hours repeatedly demonstrated the correct bat-birthing position (while imitating contractions and straining).

Finally, the labouring mother caught on and her baby was born.

But research has shown the opposite to be true. A mother who pushes *naturally* only pushes for five to six seconds, breathes once, or several times, then holds her breath and pushes again for five to six seconds.[2]

However, a mother made to push in an artificial fashion, holding her breath for 10 to 12 seconds up to three times during a contraction, often creates problems for herself and the baby. This forceful straining is referred to as a Valsalva manoeuvre in the medical literature. Here's how it works against the mother and the baby:

During sustained pushing, the pressure surrounding the mother's heart and lungs rises above normal levels. After two to three seconds of forceful pushing, this pressure reduces the amount of blood returned to her heart. Therefore, the mother's heart pumps out less blood to her body, placenta and baby. The longer she sustains the push, the more her blood pressure drops. The lower her blood pressure, the less oxygen the baby receives.[3]

This problem is compounded when the mother is lying on her back. In this position, the heavy uterus compresses the vena cava and partially obstructs the aorta. Blood flow to the mother's heart and her baby is reduced, the mother's blood pressure falls, and the uterine contractions weaken. In addition, the weight of her abdomen and uterus pushing up against her diaphragm makes breathing more difficult.

Diminished placental blood flow and decreased oxygen levels create a worrisome change in the baby's heartbeat called late decelerations. Although there are other reasons late decelerations occur, Valsalva pushing is one you can prevent. Late decelerations rightfully alarm doctors who then may want to speed delivery with forceps or a Caesarean birth. Both the remedy and prevention, however, often lie in a mother pushing naturally, in a natural position.

Along with strained and aching muscles following Valsalva pushing, many mothers report devastating psychological consequences. Zealous cheerleading often creates a feeling of desperation. A mother privately worries, "My baby will never be born," "I'm not pushing right," and finally, "It's not working, I can't do this any more." Consciously or unconsciously some mothers give up. Even if mothers succeed in this fashion, they often exaggerate the part their cheerleaders played.

Exhortations to push as hard and long as you can wrongly imply that harder pushing will lead to a faster birth.

PUSHING THE PANIC BUTTON

"As soon as I started pushing, there was hysteria in the room, everyone was frantic and screaming at me to PUSH! I thought to myself, 'Something must be wrong! They've seen lots of births— they wouldn't be acting this way if everything was okay.'

When my baby was coming out, someone asked, 'Do you want to touch him?' I said 'No' because I thought he was dead. I assumed he was dying or dead for them to be in such a panic about my pushing faster.

When he was born and laid on my belly, I was afraid to look, or to touch him." [But the baby was healthy.]

– BONNIE

NATURAL PUSHING

Once your cervix is completely open, the work and nature of labour changes. There is an unmistakable logic and harmony as this phase of birth unfolds. When women are not coached to push forcefully, they will push in the way "nature" intended.

Contractions usually slow down from every two or three minutes, to every four or five minutes, allowing you to rest after each push. A last surge of oxytocin strengthens contractions to help you push your baby out. Although you might have been "sleeping" between contractions near the end of labour, the urge to push is often accompanied by a healthy rush of adrenalin that will wake you up and get you moving for birthing and bonding with your baby.

Unlike in Valsalva pushing, during natural pushing your blood pressure and the oxygen flow to the baby fluctuate much less. Natural pushing may prolong pushing time slightly, but if you and the baby are doing well, there's no reason for concern.

When your baby has moved down deep enough into your pelvis to stretch your pelvic floor, you will feel an urge to bear down. If your baby moves down early, or if the position of his head puts pressure on those reflex points, it is possible to feel the urge to push before you are completely dilated. In most cases the cervix is soft and stretchy at this point and will dilate rapidly in response to spontaneous, short, grunty pushes at the peak of contractions.

The practice of discouraging *any* pushing until the cervix is *completely* dilated was an outgrowth of the widespread use of forceful Valsalva pushing. The goal was to prevent swelling or tearing of the cervix that may accompany Valsalva pushing, particularly if the cervix is tight. It is unfortunate that the shorter (3–4 seconds), less intense but natural, reflexive "grunts" (at the peak of contractions) are also suppressed instead of just harmful Valsalva pushing (10 seconds).

Your birth attendant can assess the elasticity of your cervix by doing a vaginal examination. If your cervix is not stretchy yet, or it's swollen, and you have the urge to push, get on your hands and knees or lie on your side. These positions reduce the pressure of the baby's head on your cervix, and decrease the overwhelming urge to push.

After you are completely dilated, contractions often slow down from every two minutes to every four to five. If the intensity of labour eases up, and you are waiting for the urge to push, you may use this time to take a shower, brush your hair and catch your second wind. The urge will come in time and you will benefit from the little break you took.

Don't be concerned if you are examined vaginally and are found to be 10 centimetres dilated but have no urge to push. This is normal. Pushing just because you are 10 centimetres, but without the urge to bear down, will be less effective and more tiring. Without vaginal examinations telling them they *should* be pushing, women will continue labouring until the urge arises.

The medical model takes a different view of the normal rest period between full dilation and the urge to push. It believes that once labour starts it can't stop or slow down. If it does, many doctors feel compelled to begin a syntocin drip, use forceps, or even perform a Caesarean.

If there is no urge to push, it's okay to wait a while. If your doctor or nurse is feeling anxious, but you and your baby are doing fine, ask for a half hour or even an hour of privacy before further action is taken. Try standing up or squatting to bring the baby deeper into your pelvis. Emptying your bladder may also help.

Occasionally the natural urge to push doesn't come, so you might begin pushing with a modified-Valsalva. Sometimes it's helpful to have your partner or birth attendant stimulate the pushing reflex by placing their fingers in your vagina and pushing downward during a contraction. This manoeuvre can "jump start" a woman's natural urge to push.

BIRTH SOUNDS

At first you may be surprised at the wonderfully primal sounds that come from your throat. Hearing those deep, grunting, growling, moaning sounds means your baby is almost born. If you tend to feel self-conscious about making noise, make sure you have made provisions for privacy. Don't let social inhibitions—yours or anyone else's—change the natural course of your birth.

> **DID YOU KNOW:**
>
> When a labouring woman squats, her pelvic outlet is 28 percent greater than in the lying-flat position!

LET GRAVITY WORK FOR YOU

Upright positions (standing, kneeling, hands-and-knees, sitting on the edge of the bed or a chair, or squatting) increase the diameter of the pelvis and strengthen uterine contractions so the baby can slide down and out. In these positions, pressure from the baby's head is applied directly and evenly to the cervix, which helps open it.

Mothers in upright positions give birth easier, faster and with less pain. In labour, move about until you find the position that helps you

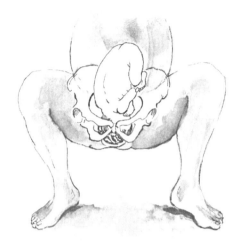

FIGURE 24.1

feel the greatest urge to push. You have to be pushing-in-awareness to find the right position for you and your baby; you can't plan this ahead of time.

In contrast to upright positions, lying on your back actually collapses the diameter of your pelvic bones a half-inch to an inch, making the passage for the baby smaller. Most mothers find this position more painful and feel they are pushing their baby uphill! As described earlier in the chapter, this position can lead to foetal distress. This type of foetal distress can be remedied by getting into an upright or side-lying position.

Figure 24.1 of a baby moving through the pelvic region of an upright-squatting mother is an example of letting gravity work for you.

BIRTHING ON YOUR BACK!? WHERE DID THIS IDEA COME FROM?

Until the late 1700s, women the world over laboured and gave birth in positions of *their* choice. They stood, sat on a birth stool, squatted, or curled up on their side. So, why has it become so common for women to give birth lying on their back when that position works against birth physiology and gravity, and is more painful for women?

Lying on a birth table was first made popular in France in 1738 by Francois Mauriceau, physician to the queen, who proposed it as an alternative to the commonly used birth chair. Mauriceau encouraged this position not because it helped women in birth, but because it facilitated *his* control of problematic delivery and the use of forceps.[4,5]

Others say it all started with King Louis XIV of France. Women in that time often gave birth sitting on a birthing chair, revealing little since they remained dressed and often were covered by a sheet. King Louis engaged his court physician to convince the ladies of the court that childbirth would be easier and simpler if they reclined on a high table. This arrangement allowed King Louis to gain sexual gratification by secretly watching the births from behind a curtain.

The immobilization of women was further advanced in 1826, when American physician William Dewees introduced stirrups to the birth table. Stirrups are metal frames and straps that support and secure a woman's legs in a wide-open position while she lies on her back (this is called lithotomy position).[6]

Technological advances also contributed to horizontal birth becoming the norm in western culture:

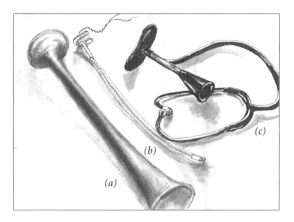

(a) First foetascope (wood).

(b) Internal foetal electrode. After the spiral wire is screwed into the baby's scalp, the guide tube is removed, and the wires are attached to a plate on the mother s leg.

(c) Modern foetascope.

The foetal stethoscope, used to listen to foetal heart tones, was invented around 1850. With this instrument, the baby's heart tones can be heard best when the mother is lying on her back because there is less movement. More and more often, even during normal deliveries, the emphasis was placed on monitoring the unborn in order to intervene if necessary. Foetal heart tones were checked frequently during the delivery, making it essential for the woman to be supine. As a result, with this advance in technology (albeit an invention of incalculable value), even women whose labour progressed without problems were delivered in a horizontal position.

At the end of the 1960s, the Doppler apparatus was invented. This instrument sends out ultrasonic signals of the unborn child's heart and converts them into sound so the foetal heart tones can be heard. With this technology, the foetal heart tones can be monitored during or between contractions while the woman is any position. Since the Doppler has replaced the foetal stethoscope, no convincing argument remains for a normal birth to take place in a horizontal position.

Naturally, transitions in standard obstetric practice cannot be expected to occur overnight. Medical information and technology alone do not destroy a deep-rooted practice of centuries.[7]

To date, most birth attendants are trained to deliver a baby with the mother on her back, with or without stirrups. Even doctors who agree upright positions are better for the mother and baby, may insist the mother lie on her back. One doctor explained his reluctance to change, "I just can't imagine how to position my hands in any position other than when the mother is lying down."

TAKE A STAND

"Stand and Deliver" isn't only suggesting the possibility of standing up when you give birth. It also means TAKE A STAND for yourself, for what you believe, and for being spontaneous in the hour you give birth. Unless there is a good reason to do otherwise, stand up for the birth sounds and position that are right for you.

BIRTH POSITIONS

One of the following positions may turn out to be the best for you. In our classes, parents become familiar with these positions by trying each of them out.

HANDS-AND-KNEES

This position allows you full range of motion in your hips; rocking can feel good during contractions. Between contractions you can lean forward and rest on your partner, a big bean bag, birthing ball or pile of pillows.

Hands-and-knees position is especially useful in "back labour," so named because the pain of contractions is felt more in the lower back than in the cervix. Back labour occurs when the baby is lying face-up (looking at the pubis). This is also called "sunny side up," or posterior position. In this position the back of a baby's head pushes on the mother's sacrum.

When a mother having back labour lies on her back, the pain becomes unbearable as the baby's head pushes hard against her sacrum during contractions. Lying flat on her back will not only slow (or stop) cervical dilation, but may also prevent the rotation of

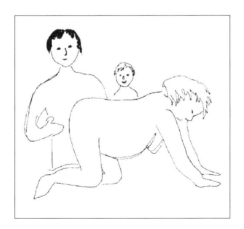

"I imagine giving birth on my hands and knees. My husband will help me, and my daughter wants to be there, too."

JULIA DESCRIBES HER DRAWING

the baby's head to a face-down position. This is one cause of "posterior arrest," which doctors may try to correct with syntocin, epidurals, forceps or a Caesarean birth.

There is another solution. It's simple physics: if a mother is on her hands and knees, the weight of the baby's body and head may fall downward towards the mother's belly and make for an easier birth. It's good to keep in mind that even if a baby does not turn, if labour continues to progress, it can be born "sunny side up."

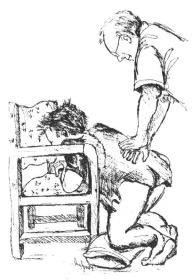

A partner or midwife can ease lower back pain with the welcome sensation of a heating pad, hot or cold compresses, deep massage of the hips or sustained lumbar counter-pressure.

KNEELING

From hands and knees you can easily move into the kneeling position. With soft pillows under your knees, lean on a chair, bed, or your partner when you push or rest between contractions.

SITTING

Sitting on the edge of a chair or your bed provides the benefits of gravity and the comfort of support. You can lean into your birth companion for extra support.

SQUATTING

Women the world over push and give birth in the squatting position. In between contractions women rest their legs, stand, stretch, kneel, or sit back on a foot stool.

Since squatting is easier for women who are already used to it, begin integrating squatting into your daily life. Squat when you peel potatoes or do garden work. If it's difficult to keep your balance, try leaning against a wall, back-to-back against your partner, or squatting over your partner's thighs. Once you've practiced, you may be able to hold a squat for five minutes.

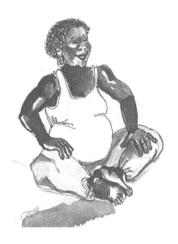

The Butterfly exercise helps stretch inner thigh muscles in preparation for opening up or squatting to push out your baby. Push the soles of your feet together and gently press your knees towards the floor. Gradually move your heels towards your perineum to increase the stretch in your groin. See where you feel the stretch when you lean backwards or forwards.

STANDING

Standing allows you to really open your legs wide and lower yourself into each push. It also relieves back pressure and lets you stretch out or walk around.

You can lean your back against your partner, and hang freely from his strong arms under your arms. Or you can face each other and hold on to his shoulders or grasp his arms.

Here's how one mother envisioned her position in labour, both physically and spiritually (Figure 24.2).

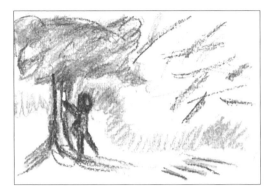

FIGURE 24.2 "I made a stickfigure—but it s a fat stick figure. I am leaning on a tree which is [representing] Nature. I have a feeling I will need to stand up to get my baby out. The brown lines [lower right] is life flowing out of me. The colourful strokes [upper right] is my fear. The yellow [body halo] is protection, it's God keeping the fear out."

SAMARA

ON THE TOILET

Sitting on the toilet naturally is associated with the physical release of your perineum. During birthing it can be a good place for psychological release, as well as for privacy and making use of gravity. Periodic checks by your midwife or nurse will allow you plenty of time to give birth elsewhere.

LYING ON YOUR BACK

Although lying flat on your back would be unusual, it could be the birthing position that feels just right for you. If this is the case, do it! However, if this position is suggested by someone else and it doesn't feel like it's working, try another position.

DON'T PULL BACK ON YOUR THIGHS if you are pushing in a semi-sitting position or lying on your back. It's hard to push down and pull back at the same time. Let your helpers hold your legs up for you. You have enough work to do.

AVOID THE LITHOTOMY POSITION. This unnatural position is advantageous only to the doctor (Figure 24.3). When a mother's legs are

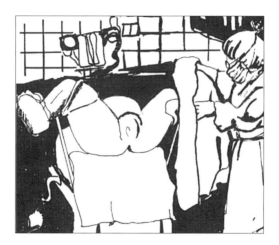

FIGURE 24.3 Lithotomy Position. "The vulva, perineum, and adjacent regions have been thoroughly scrubbed. The *field* is sterile, draped in preparation for delivery [emphasis added]."[8]

It is worthwhile to note that the nurse is active while the birthing mother is passive. Also, note that this common depiction of birth, in which the mother is without face, reduces her to an object, "a scrubbed perineum," a "field," *something* to be delivered.

spread wide open and flexed back on stirrups, her perineum becomes unnaturally taut and is more likely to tear or "need" an episiotomy.

Stirrups also may cause painful cramping, numbness, or blood clots in the legs. In addition, some women experience this position as degrading, vulnerable and powerless.

ROPES

A doctor at the University of New Mexico Hospital told me he attended a Navajo woman on the reservation. She grasped a strong rope hanging from the ceiling in her *hogan* (traditional Navajo dwelling) and lowered herself into a squat as she pushed.

Many women find they push better when they are "hanging" or pulling downward into a squat from a high mantle, buffet, window sill or their birth partner's arms.

HAMMOCK

A woman in one of my childbirth classes described a birth-hammock she observed when living in El Salvador. A large piece of cloth is stretched between two big rocks, and held in place by the weight of other rocks. The birthing mother squats over the hammock and her child is born into the soft cloth.

*

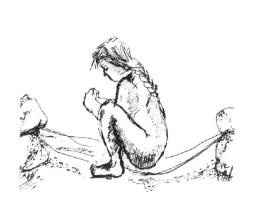

EPISIOTOMY EPIDEMIC

Ninety percent of women who give birth attended by doctors get an episiotomy.[9] This figure is in sharp contrast to the ten percent incidence of episiotomy among women attended by midwives. The high rate of episiotomy use among doctors is most likely caused by several factors:

1. Few doctors have learned how to deliver a baby over an intact perineum, and most are reluctant to try something new.
2. They lack the faith or patience to wait the additional five or ten minutes for the baby's head to emerge slowly on its own.
3. Delivery positions favoured by doctors tend to make episiotomy more necessary.

4. Many doctors base their decision to perform routine episiotomy on a notion that episiotomy prevents damage to the birth canal. Yet, research has not been able to to support that idea.

5. Use of epidurals increases forceps use, which requires an episiotomy.

6. Doctors' belief in the *need* for episiotomy is reinforced by their not realizing that many of the perineal tears they've seen were attributable to frantic, well-meaning exhortations to PUSH! during crowning, and lithotomy position, rather than to women's anatomical weakness.

PROTECTING YOUR PERINEUM DURING BIRTH

Natural pushing will increase the likelihood of birthing your baby over an intact perineum (without episiotomy or tearing). Here's a few general tips to help protect your perineum:

• Kegel throughout pregnancy to improve vaginal tone, and increase your conscious awareness of that muscle (see Chapter 42).

• Know your birth attendant's philosophy regarding natural pushing, restrictions on pushing time, and "acceptable" positions.

• Avoid lithotomy position or pulling back on your legs (which tightens the perineum).

• Consider the side-lying position, which helps bring about a slow birth and the fewest perineal tears.

TIPS FOR THE "HOME-STRETCH":

This moment-to-moment direction and encouragement helps the mother connect and cooperate with her body. As soon as the baby's head emerges, the ring-of-fire immediately subsides and the baby is quickly born.

WHAT TO DO WHEN YOUR BABY IS CROWNING

1. When your baby's head begins to show, your partner or your
    attendant can apply warm wet washcloths to your perineum.
    Keep a big basin, bowl, or crockpot full of very warm water
    or ginger tea water. Don't wring the washcloths too dry—a
    little moisture feels better. Firm, steady counter-pressure on
    the perineum and anus brings welcome relief during
    contractions. This is especially true the few moments before
    the head is born, soothing the burning sensation women refer
    to as the "ring of fire." (Discard washcloths soiled with
    blood or little bits of stool normally excreted with pushing.)
2. Before you are in labour, ask your midwife, partner or
    doctor to tell you when your baby's head is crowning
    (staying in full view between contractions). At this time
    begin pushing gently in short (3 second), grunty pushes. This
    will ease your baby's head out slowly, a quarter inch at a
    time, over your stretchy perineum. It is also helpful to
    continue pushing gently *between* contractions, without the
    extra force of uterine pressure.

    You and your partner can agree on a cue word for this
    gentle pushing, such as "Baby pushes," "Gentle pushes,"
    "Little grunts," or "Easy does it." Hearing that special
    phrase will remind you instantly what you need to do. Kind
    encouragement spoken slowly and softly often is
    appreciated. You might like to hear, "Open to our baby,"
    "The baby is coming, don't hold back, it's okay, it's
    time ... "
3. When your baby's head is crowning, lubricating the
    perineum with K-Y jelly or oil will help your baby slide out.

    Any unscented vegetable oil will do; it's more convenient
    to use in a small bottle. Use at room temperature, or warm
    it up in the hot water being used for perineal compresses.

    Some mothers like perineal massage at this time, others
    don't. It's only useful if you like it. While perineal massage
    may feel good, there's no evidence that it actually prevents
    tearing.

4. When your baby's head is crowning, *reach down and feel
    your baby's head emerging.* This is a wonderful moment to
    feel one with your baby and your body. Feeling your thinned-
    out perineum stretching over your baby's slowly emerging
    head with each push tells you just how gently to push!
5. I tell a father to use his most tender voice to guide the
    mother, telling her what he is seeing (her eyes are usually
    closed as she must focus intensely inward). As she pushes
    gently, he encourages her, saying,

"I see a little more hair ..."
And she pushes gently again, listening for his report,
"I see the forehead coming out,"
She gives a gentle push ...
"now the eyes,"
Another gentle push,
"the nose,"
The last little push,
"oooh the mouth ... you did it! ... The baby's head is turning now
... okay, another medium push and our baby will be born ..."

Chapter 25

How To Give Birth *If You Need a Caesarean*

When I was pregnant, I always skipped over the chapters on Caesareans … I was sure that would never happen to me.

THE POWER OF CAESAREAN-SEMANTICS

When the subject of Caesarean sections comes up in class, I ask expectant parents the following question: "What comes to mind when you hear the words 'C-Section' or 'Sectioned?'"

Their immediate responses include:

- "knife"
- "I'm not part of the birth"
- "blood"
- "… having it done *to* me"
- "being cut open"
- "… being a helpless observer"
- "losing control"
- "loneliness"
- "fear"
- "disappointment"

I also see non-verbal responses: grimaces, hunched up shoulders and tension in their bodies.

*

THE FIRST CAESAREAN ... AND VBAC!

"The one thing we know absolutely about the Caesarean section in ancient times is that it was not performed on Aurelia at the birth of her son, Julius, later Julius Caesar. He arrived in quite the usual manner. The misunderstanding came about because in seventh century (B.C.) Rome, one Numa Pompilius decreed that if a woman died while pregnant, the child was instantly to be cut out of her abdomen. This dictum was part of the *Lex Regia*, and was later incorporated into the *Lex Caesare*, from which the operation acquired the label 'Caesarean section.'

The first record of a successful Caesarean [the mother also survived] comes much later when in the year 1500 the wife of Jacob Nufer, a Swiss sowgelder, went into labour and could not seem to deliver ... In his desperation Nufer at least knew where to begin.

Thirteen midwives (so the story goes) had tried and failed, at which point Jacob collected his tools of the trade and did the obvious. Is it possible he had the intuition to clean them first? To wash his hands? To protect his wife from the barnyard flies? We will simply never know. All that is apparent is that at the operation's close, both mother and child were doing well. In fact, Mom Nufer did very well indeed. In time she gave birth to six more children, including twins, all of whom she delivered normally. She lived to the fine age of seventy-seven."

– NANCY CALDWELL SOREL
EVER SINCE EVE[1]

Then I ask, "Suppose I say 'Caesarean-Birth,' or 'You're going to give *birth* by Caesarean,' what images or feelings come up?"

After quiet reflection, people say things like:

- It's better ... l feel like I'm still part of what's happening."
- "... the baby still needs me to be there, to welcome it, to nurse it ..."
- "I feel less like a failure."
- "I'm seeing the baby, not an operating room."

- "I feel like a mother—not just a body the doctors are working on …"
- "I feel less scared."

This question generates different non-verbal messages, too: softening of the body and facial expressions, pensive looks, smiles, and sighs of relief.

Parents leave this exercise in the Power of Caesarean-Semantics with an image of Caesarean as a birth, not a C-section. I also suggest they remind those who lack this consciousness to refer to a Caesarean-section as Caesarean-birth. It makes a huge difference to see yourself (or another woman) as a mother who gave birth, rather than as someone who was "sectioned."

Caesarean-Semantics also examines two acronyms that refer to mothers who've had a previous Caesarean. The first is VBAC, (Vaginal Birth After Caesarean) and the second is TOLAC (*Trial* of Labour After Caesarean).

When mothers and their birth attendants use VBAC, they are more likely to envision a normal birth. On the other hand, TOLAC, which has become widely used in recent years, conjures up images of uncertainty, failure and even guilt.

GRIEVING THE DISRUPTED RITE OF PASSAGE

When Ellen told friends she'd had a C-section, they asked, "What went *wrong*?" (rather than inquiring about the birth). Their conversations became technological post-mortems which left Ellen feeling alienated and confused. She struggled with doubts about whether she could have, or should have, prevented her Caesarean. Her experience of having given birth faded into the background.

It's difficult for the average friend or relative to strike a balance between acknowledging what the (Caesarean) mother went through and missed out on, while helping her celebrate her birth. The mother and her friends need to recognize that the baby's birth and the mother's "birth" are separate events. Even though mother and baby are healthy (that's the most important thing), a disrupted transition into motherhood can have a profound impact on the family's future, particularly if the mother's loss is ignored or discounted.

For some mothers who've gone through an unexpectedly difficult

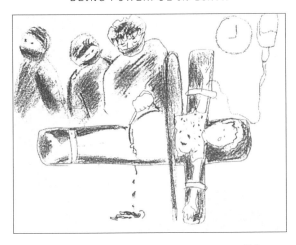

Jane's drawing of her Caesarean birth: "I felt cut off from giving birth. I did not feel the birth or feel like I gave birth."

labour or Caesarean birth, the feelings of not being in control or of having failed at giving birth undermine their maternal confidence. I've seen this loss of confidence expressed as postpartum depression, anger, problematic infant-bonding and inadequate care of the baby. In addition, marital stress often results when a husband is unable to understand or empathize with his wife's emotional pain. Timely counselling may be crucial, not only for women, but for their husbands as well.

As is the case with other losses, grieving is an essential part of healing. Without permission and encouragement to grieve, wounded parents remain burdened by their invisible pain.

A WOMAN DOES NOT GIVE BIRTH IN A VOID

When people asked me why I had a Caesarean, I didn't know how to answer. I now realize how unmanageably complex that question is, and that I'll never know the answer. Yet at the time, I thought understanding what had happened would help me regain control. My zealous search spanned years before pushing my consciousness to a paradoxical place of understanding while not-knowing.

Here's what I've come to believe: *In the moment a Caesarean birth (or any event) happens, no one can know all the forces which converged to create that event.*

As Kaarin became aware that her baby would need to be born by Caesarean, she felt swept away with feelings of frustration, failure, and unfocused anger; she had given every ounce of herself and it wasn't enough. Yet, part of her was relieved that the ordeal was coming to an end.

In that moment, holding her birth-power sculpture, Kaarin reached deep within herself to a place she hadn't even known existed, gritted her teeth, and renewed her commitment to *be* at her baby's Caesarean-birth.

Almost simultaneously, her husband leaned over and whispered softly, "You've been so strong—I'm so proud of how brave you've been. I love you. We're going to do this together."

Kaarin and her husband, in their cocoon of love, birthed their baby in the cold, bright operating room.

Labour and birth unfold within a
complex, and infinite web,
Spun by the mother,
And by everyone who has ever taught her
about mothering, birth, sexuality, pain,
control and surrender.
All the people at her birth
helped spin the web with threads from
their histories, beliefs, experiences, fears …
and recent birth experiences that they have witnessed,
which empowered or terrified them.

CROSS THE RIVER NO BLAME—I CHING

So, no single decision, no one doctor, and no mother is solely responsible for a birth outcome. It's over-simplified to blame or praise any individual or isolated event for how a birth turns out. Our challenge is to live with ambiguity, embrace the birth that happened, and move on with our family into its future.

THE CAESAREAN NEXUS

> Nex'us, *n* [L. from pp. of *nectere*, to bind] A connection, tie, or link between individuals of a group, members of a series, etc.

Fueled by economic incentives and defensive medicine prompted by fears of costly litigation, the Caesarean-birth rate peaked in the US in the early eighties and continued at high levels (25–30 percent) until 1990 when the rate began to drop. This encouraging trend partially reflects heightened medical and consumer awareness that Caesarean births are not automatic solutions to deviations from the obstetric norm.

However, the most direct pressure to lower the rate of Caesarean births has come from the explosion of managed healthcare. Expensive, surgical births are no longer lucrative—within managed care they are threats to the corporate "bottom line."

STACEY'S VBAC STORY

Stacey, a 34 year-old mother and nurse, was having her first baby. She was knowledgeable about birth and how routine intervention could change the course of a normal labour. With that in mind, she approached her doctor in an effort to reach an agreement to avoid routine monitoring, IV, and bed rest in labour. Stacey's doctor gave vague reassurances while sending a disapproving message to her that she was "making your birth experience more important than the life of your baby." (The reality that prenatal care and birth can be low-tech and fulfilling *without* risking the baby's health is overlooked routinely.)

Like many women, Stacey became uncomfortable and anxious about pursuing the issue. She considered changing doctors, but wanted to avoid an upsetting confrontation. She went on to rationalize that "as long as my baby is okay, it doesn't matter what I have to go through."

During labour, she continued to minimize the cumulative impact routine interventions were having, saying to herself, "Well, what's a little IV? What's a little pitocin [called syntocin in the UK]? My body is stronger than all this." However:

THE BITTER TASTE OF COURTROOM MEDICINE

"Dr. Leo Cooper [not his real name], an OB/GYN at one of Manhattan's most prestigious hospitals, sat in a downtown courtroom as a jury heard about a child he had delivered eight years before who was normal at birth but was diagnosed eight months later with a muscular weakness on one side of his body. Cooper was accused of having missed the symptoms of fetal distress—which he claims were not present—and therefore not having performed a cesarean section. After a three-week trial—with the young boy sitting in the courtroom, one arm hanging at his side—Cooper was found negligent.

'I'm 46,' he says, 'and I'm very cynical. Nobody wants to deliver babies, because they feel that regardless of what they do and how they do it, they are judged by the outcome, and the judgment is by show: Who puts on the best show?

At my trial, they had an OB for their side who's testified as a witness at least 200 times. I'd never been in a courtroom before ... You're not sure who to dislike more, the lawyers for putting on this show or the doctors who come and lie on the stand.'

Cooper is still delivering babies—at least for now. 'The people I work with all happen to enjoy doing obstetrics,' he says. 'You have the ability to do something positive and constructive, and it makes you feel good about yourself. This stuff doesn't make you feel less good about yourself, but it makes you look at all your patients as potential adversaries. You come back to the office and see people sitting there smiling at you, and all you can see is the other people in the courtroom with daggers. It sours you.'"

– AIMEE LEE BALL
NEW YORK MAGAZINE

One concession led to another. First the IV, then the pitocin. Strapped to a monitor I had to lie on my back. The pain became intolerable after the pitocin, so I had an epidural, which made my blood pressure drop—which stressed my baby—so I had to have oxygen and lots of IV fluids. I couldn't feel the urge to pee, so the nurses catheterized me four times. I couldn't feel my contractions so I couldn't push right, and in the end I had a Caesarean I *know* was unnecessary. I should have stood up to that doctor in his office.

A year later Stacey came to see me because she was struggling with depression, self-doubt and feelings of loss. She frequently berated herself for "taking so long to get over having a Caesarean."

I suggested she make a picture depicting her most vivid memory of the Caesarean birth and bring it to our next session. I include Stacey's watercolour (Figure 25.1) and her comments about it to illustrate the complex process of self-discovery that can be triggered through the use of birth art:

> It is a tortured, ugly picture of birth. The doctor is as big as the knife. But the bloody knife is dominant, it's what your eye sees first [ladle-like shape].
>
> There is a bright light hanging overhead … an empty labour bed that looks like a grave. It might be empty because I "left" (emotionally) during labour to escape the pitocin-pain and the feeling of helplessness.
>
> The nurses [three female signs with legs at the nurses' station] stand over me and are in the way. I wanted to believe in myself in spite of all their interventions. But none of them ever told me I could do it.
>
> The woman is me, the circle inside is my baby.

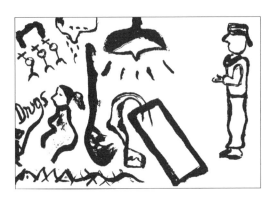

FIGURE 25.1

[When Stacey realized she hadn't given herself arms or legs, she remembered feeling helpless and childlike in the hospital, and began to cry.]

The yellow circle in front of me represents the four times I was catheterized after the epidural. "Drugs" is scrawled in red. The "g" is meant to be the IV trailing down into me.

Beneath me is a wavy black line which is the motion of labour … but it is hatched with barbed wire and spotted with blood.

That's my husband [to the left of the light on top] looking down. Those are tears falling as he watches what happened. He was concerned and disappointed in the way I gave birth, but he didn't really cry. So this part of my painting doesn't make sense to me.

My husband is logical in day-to-day life and indifferent when I talk or cry about my disappointment in the birth. Maybe he doesn't understand because he is a man, or because he has bought into the medical model's definition of a "good" birth—a birth that results in a healthy baby. I think my being upset about what happened scares him.

In therapy, and with the support of other women, Stacey slowly regained her confidence in her body's ability to birth normally. Two years later, pregnant with her second child, Stacey hired a birth attendant who respected her desire to have a low-intervention, normal birth. Her second daughter was born, without drugs, after six hours of active labour. Stacey finally experienced what she had known all along, that her body knew how to give birth.

DOES FOETAL ASPHYXIA IN LABOUR CAUSE BRAIN DAMAGE?

Evidence shows that "asphyxia is far more likely to be the result of … prenatal influences such as genetics, toxic exposures, infection [and inadequate diet]. When under 5% of babies with very low five-minute Apgar scores (0–3) show any subsequent neurologic damage, and only 15% of children with cerebral palsy have a history of very low Apgars, the hypothetical connection between asphyxia and neurologic impairment is clearly in question."

– LEAH ALBERS, CNM, DrPh
CHILDBIRTH INSTRUCTOR MAGAZINE[3]

A few weeks later, I visited Stacey and asked her to use birth art to portray her second birth (Figure 25.2). Stacey was happy and excited as she described her picture:

> This time I birthed normally, so what first came to mind was an image of my baby's head coming out of my vagina [black oval surrounded by a bold red ring]. This is me in labour, leaning into a rocking chair [above and to the right of the inner red ring]. The black wavy line [under her] is the pain. Pain was not such a big deal, but it was there!
>
> Three guardian angels [lower right, with pretty coloured wings] were with me in labour—these were my sister, friend and midwife.
>
> During the birth, my husband was sitting in the rocking chair and I knelt into him [lower left]. Men have that solid, physical, muscular strength. When I was tired and pushing, I tapped into his strength. It helped a lot having him there.
>
> Here is the three of us right after our daughter's birth [upper left]. Giving birth *normally* has had an unexpected, positive impact on our marriage, too. My husband says he sees me differently, now he thinks of me as *strong*. I, also, realized my strength and power by giving birth, and am bringing those qualities to our marriage.
>
> The left upper corner was coloured black to symbolize the painful aspects of my first birth. The pain and pleasure of birth are part of the human drama. Contemplating and resolving what happened during the Caesarean birth was an important part of this birth, and it will always be a part of me.

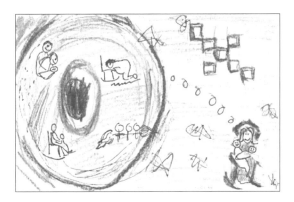

FIGURE 25.2 Stacey's drawing of her home birth

I believe that things happen randomly but that there's a pattern, there is order in chaos [red and green boxes]. Now I see a pattern in all that happened in my births—how my beliefs and self-image somehow meshed with each of my birth experiences.

The jewels [yellow "stars"] are the insights I've gotten from my Caesarean birth and everything in between. All of the gems are helping me be a better mother.

The lightly-coloured shading over the picture is the fabric that holds this whole experience together. Both birth experiences are a part of my whole life, and they affect my daughters, too. It's not just MY experience, it's their experience, too.

WHAT TO DO AT A CAESAREAN BIRTH:

- Encourage everyone to call it a Caesarean birth.
- Focus on thoughts about giving birth and welcoming your baby; don't let the surgical preparations distract you.

DADS:

- Overcome your understandable intimidation (or fascination) by the operating room. Sit close to mum and hold her (everything *behind* the blue curtain is a sterile field, but her head and shoulders will welcome your reassuring touch).
- Ask the doctor or nurse to cue you when the baby is emerging. Peek over the curtain and watch your baby be born—describe the baby to the mother ("It has black hair," "fat cheeks," "bright eyes," etc.).
- Sometimes, a cooperative anaesthesiologist will lower the curtain for a moment so the mum can watch the birth!
- Understand that a Caesarean-born baby has to go to the warmer for a few minutes after birth. If you can see the baby, tell the mum what it's doing so she can feel connected, too.
- After the baby is swaddled, lay it on the mother's chest so she can see, smell, and cuddle it.

Chapter 26

Being at a Birth Doesn't Make a Man a Father

> When my son was born, I was excited, but also felt a hint of disappointment, emptiness, and guilt. I'd hoped the miracle of birth would overwhelm and transform me, and connect me to my deepest emotions. But that didn't quite happen. Nor did I feel a flash of instant, intense bonding from being there to see him born. But later, after years of adoring and caring for my little boy, the memory of his birth was infused with the love which I had come to feel. It was those years of fathering which finally made the memory of my son's birth so powerful.
>
> ROB HOROWITZ

The forces which expanded the father's role in birth unfortunately caused some parents to believe that his new role would ensure or increase his involvement with childrearing. Anxious mothers have confided to me their concern that if the father is not at the birth (or intensely involved), he will have missed the critical opportunity for bonding with the baby.

Witnessing the drama of birth may have a profound emotional effect on some fathers. Nevertheless, the degree and intensity of a father's participation in birth doesn't necessarily determine the quality of his future parenting.

There are some situations, whether because of the father's temperament or stress in the couple's relationship, where the father's presence at birth may be emotionally painful to the mother, and even disrupt the course of labour. After all, giving birth is a vulnerable and intimate experience, which requires trust in oneself and in those who are there to provide support.

In these circumstances the mother should consider who she *wants* to attend her during labour. This may mean saying "No" to the baby's father, but a woman can do it if she prepares, and gets support.

Some women fear that blocking the father from being at the labour will create additional problems in their relationship. Sadly, there are some troubled men for whom any limit set by a woman triggers confrontation or rage.

One possible compromise is to labour without the father, but invite him to witness the birth of his child and to help with newborn care. These situations are awkward and difficult. Each mother has to decide what her priority is, and what choice is best for her.

SECTION V

Fathers and Birth Companions

Chapter 27

Getting Dads Involved

Not so long ago I attended a birth for the first time since my own. To breathe with the mother, to watch the child's head appear, to experience the entire process moment by moment allowed me to touch a primordial element in my being. I laughed, and cried, experienced fear, empathetic pain, and deep joy. I was standing at the doorway of existence, feeling, as deeply as I had ever felt, the connectedness of my humanity to the rest of nature with her cycles of spring and winter, creation and decay.

RAM DASS

FROM INTRODUCTION TO *WHO DIES?* BY STEPHEN LEVINE

HISTORICAL PERSPECTIVE: HOW FATHERS ENTERED THE BIRTH ROOM

Most fathers anticipate with warmth and excitement the birth of their child. But they frequently struggle with what role they should play at their baby's birth (and as a father). After all, the twentieth century saw dramatic swings in what being a father means in our culture.

Historically, fathers have been peripheral to women giving birth. Most of our grandfathers were not invited into the birth room—nor did most want to be there. Birth was considered women's business. After the midwife or doctor arrived at the home (often brought by the father), fathers puttered about in the shed, fixed household items or protected the birth place by ensuring privacy for his labouring wife.

One father recalled how his grandmother, who had eight children on an Iowa farm, always laboured with only the help of a woman relative. After the first birth, his grandfather knew it was his job to take the older children to town so his wife could labour in peace and quiet.

When the birthplace shifted from home to hospital, the custom of excluding fathers and visitors (including women) from the birth room continued. Unfortunately, hospitals underestimated the profoundly positive influence provided by the constant presence of a caring woman friend, relative, doula or midwife. Replacing this kind of support from women with nurses too busy to stay at the bedside, and with whom the mother had no prior connection, made birth an unnecessarily lonely and terrifying experience.

Meanwhile, the father went home, back to work or paced a rut in the waiting room carpet, waiting for the announcement of his child's birth. Until recently, men had only vague notions about what happened in labour and birth.

*

In America in the 1970s two developments dramatically influenced the role of fathers in the birth place. The first was the desire by couples for fathers to take a greater role in childrearing than was the case in previous generations.

The second were the birthing classes initiated by Fernand Lamaze and Robert Bradley. Instead of bringing back the doula (professional birth companion) to reduce the labouring mothers' isolation and fear during birth, the classes promoted a new role for fathers.

For the first time fathers, instead of women experienced with birth, were given the responsibility of helping mothers through childbirth. The term "labour coach" became part of the English language. As a result, fathers sought, and/or were expected to play, a larger role than they had ever had in history.

*

CONNECTING WITH OTHER FATHERS

Even though fathers have re-entered the birth room, many still feel "invisible" at childbirth classes, as well as during prenatal visits and labour. Yet, for fathers to be emotionally present at the birth of their child, they need support to clarify their role and to have their concerns validated.

In Birthing From Within classes, fathers and birth companions get special time to do this. I set aside part of one childbirth class to allow them to talk with each other about their hopes, expectations and fears. (During this time the mothers enjoy talking with each other while working on an art or writing project in another room.)

Men relish the chance to talk with other fathers about their private worries: how they will respond to their wives' pain; the responsibility of participating in important medical decisions (especially the use of pain medications or an epidural); the possibility that the baby may not be healthy at birth; and impending changes in their marriage and finances. They often reflect on their own relationship with their father, and try to imagine what fathering will be like.

I also encourage fathers to talk to men they know who have become fathers. Just as mothers-to-be can learn so much from women who've been through childbirth, fathers-to-be can be enlightened by the feelings and experiences of men they like and respect.

Guys (being guys) don't typically initiate this kind of emotional, personal sharing. But when they're asked to talk about the birth of their child, they often become animated and emotional.

The following questions are examples of things you might want to ask fathers who've been through it:

- What was most moving about the birth?
- What was surprising or scary?
- What was your first thought when you saw your baby?
- Did you cut the cord?
- What do wish you had known beforehand?

This kind of "research" is part of what expectant fathers can do for their own childbirth preparation.

*

FATHERS' BIRTH ART

When I first began introducing making-birth-art as a learning process in childbirth classes, I assumed fathers would not want to participate. I was wrong. Fathers did not hesitate to grab crayons and pastels and get right to work on their images.

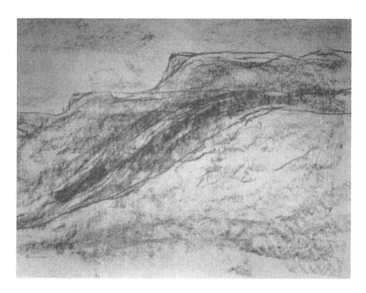

FIGURE 27.1

Typically, mothers and fathers make their own drawings, but sometimes a couple works together. In the latter case, one partner describes the image to the other who is designated the "artist."

Couples have fun seeing each other's artwork. Intuitive learning and expansion of ideas flourish during this process. Fathers are eager to share their artwork and insights.

In one class I suggested couples make a picture of the *Journey/Landscape of Birth*. Chip used pastels to make a river running through a gorge (Figure 27.1). Water, the river, represents the movement of labour, and although it appears to be going upstream he intended it to be moving through the gorge. Having few expectations or fears about birthing, Chip was open to all the possibilities labour could offer. He was absolutely excited about the upcoming birth of his child.

*

Patrick, a family-practice doctor, was eager to use birth art to help prepare for birth from the heart. He made the following drawings during several sessions.

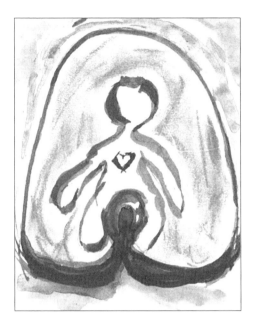

FIGURE 27.2

Pat's *Pregnant Woman* (Figure 27.2) in watercolour depicts his pregnant wife in a transcendent birth symmetry: "She is at once giving birth to the earth and being birthed by the earth. She is in a 'womb,' and being born as a mother."

When asked to make a picture reflecting his thoughts on the birth of a father, of himself as father, he stared pensively at his paper for a while before saying softly, "Probably in most cultures the focus is on the mother in pregnancy. There are lots of symbols for mother, but with father ... suddenly, there is a loss of symbols."

He reached for a paint brush and began watercolouring *Birth of a Father* (Figure 27.3). As he finished this drawing in pastels, Patrick mused sadly:

I felt real alone yesterday as a father. If I try to talk to other fathers about "fathering" or the changes or emotions I'm feeling about becoming a father—men refer to the [concrete] situation or econom-ics, not their *feelings*.

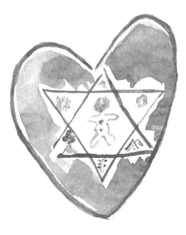

FIGURE 27.3

I asked myself, *"What* am I afraid of?"* I'm afraid of losing *the tie* or connection I have with Lisa. Our relationship is already changing, and will continue to change. I think I'm grieving the loss of what Lisa and I have shared together until now. But I'm supposed to be strong and support her.

The [blue and green] triangles represents the trinity in each of us. The birth is coming from the two of us. The blue flower, yellow dandelion and cactus are female symbols. The male symbols, mountains and a pine tree, are reaching upward and the life spring [blue scribble in top triangle]—represents my search for finding my life source. Who am I as a father? Not what should I *do*, but how to *be*? If I'm supporting Lisa, the birth and a family, then what's supporting or feeding me?

The pink baby in the middle is not a girl, I just saw a pink baby. Its cord [the red dot] is tied to my heart.

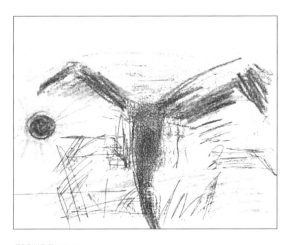

FIGURE 27.4

Lee, a first-time father drew Figure 27.4 in pastels. He called his drawing *My Journey to Fatherhood and My Child's Journey Through Birth*. Lee thoughtfully explained his drawing:

> The mouth of the cave is nestled in the mountains. There is a stream coming out of the cliff, into the green earth.
>
> The mountains represent strength. The cliffs are the transition between what was dark and closed into what is open and light.
>
> The water … stream is symbolic for purity coming into light, life, warmth—becoming alive, opening up to life.
>
> This picture is about my journey and the child's journey through birth; my journey out of darkness and the child's out of darkness, the womb.

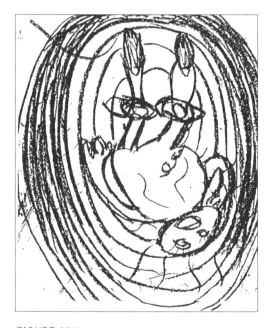

FIGURE 27.5

In his colourful, pastel drawing of *Womb With A View* (Figure 27.5) Tod, a first-time expectant father, poetically expressed his deepening connection with his growing baby, his gestation as a father, and awe at the mother-child relationship:

> I drew the [brown] concentric circles around the baby to illustrate the almost hypnotic effect the pregnancy and baby have had on me. While in utero the baby is very much a part of Alecia and I feel like much of what the baby knows of me is through Alecia's feelings, voice, and even thoughts. So, I drew the [blue] umbilical cord into Alecia's eyes, which are part of the baby's body. Recently, I've begun to feel the baby's developing personality which I showed with the bright [red] lines around her eyes. The baby wears an expression of constant amazement and curiosity, much like I feel during this pregnancy.
>
> [Tod drew Alecia's hair around the oval "face" that is seeing their baby.]

Helping fathers express their emotional depth and understand their protective role in birth is another way this approach encourages a *family's* birth from within.

Chapter 28

Pitfalls of Labour Coaching

My wife did great in labour. I don't know what she would have done without me.

PROUD, BUT GRANDIOSE, NEW DAD

Witnessing a woman giving birth is a profoundly moving human experience. A father should be supported and encouraged to just be there, to soak up the miracle of his child's birth.

Fathers bring reassurance, protection and love to the mother of their child. One of the tenets of the Birthing From Within approach is that a father offers much more as a partner than as a "coach."

It's sad that fathers have been burdened by the idea that their "coaching" is central to labour's success. While this is an unfair position to put fathers in, it can be damaging to women as well.

Once a woman believes she needs to be "coached," she is alienated from her instinctive core, where the strength and confidence necessary for birthing wait to be tapped. She may become more dependent

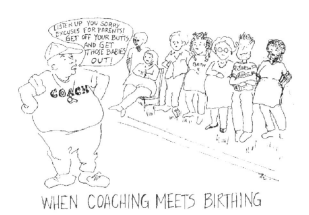

WHEN COACHING MEETS BIRTHING

on her coach or technology than on her own resources. That kind of passivity is contrary to doing the hard work required in labour.

The idea of playing "coach" to their wives makes a lot of men squirm; they sense that labour coaching can get them into trouble in a couple of ways. First, the coach runs the risk of becoming a scapegoat if labour is more difficult or painful than expected (and the breathing-relaxation techniques don't bring the hoped-for relief and control).

When the going gets rough in labour, some coaches try harder to get a mother to "relax," or make progress. Ironically, excessive support and encouragement may increase the mother's performance anxiety and lead to feelings of shame and failure on her part. While in some situations stuck labour *causes* anxiety (in the mother and in others), in other situations it is *anxiety* which is a critical factor in causing a stuck labour.

On the other hand, if the birth has gone smoothly, the coach may be given, or take, undue credit for the positive outcome. Mothers in these circumstances have confided to me that they resented how their own efforts were minimized. In either case, marital discord can be an unfortunate outcome of fathers entering the "coaching" business.

"I feel the most important thing the birthing woman does is to listen to her own body and find out what her body is telling her she needs to do. And that neither the partner, nor the midwife, nor the doula, or whomever, should be giving orders, 'Now do this' or 'Now do that' because that interferes with what she is really trying to get from her body. The coach image is the guy who's standing there telling the player what to do—the coach is up here and the player down there somewhere."

– MARSDEN WAGNER, M.D.[1]

Chapter 29

What's a Father to Do?

A calm, watchful, loving presence protects the fragile harmony
of birth; frantic coaching has never been part of nature's plan.

Birthing From Within classes encourage fathers to be present in a
loving, gentle way, supporting the mother by sensing her needs and
offering suggestions, not directives. It's not so much what you know
or what you do that makes a difference, it's just being there and
believing in her.

Here are a few tips I share with fathers and birth companions to
help them escape their dilemma about what to do:

BE YOURSELF

A father can only *do* so much at the actual birth. Being present and
supportive is perhaps the best we can hope for—and you accomplish
this in your own way—maybe just holding her hand, rubbing her
back, putting a cold washcloth on her head. You don't need to know
about birth, just love her.

JAKE, FATHER OF FOUR

Couples who are affectionate and touch a lot before labour, for example, will naturally continue to do so during labour. It stands to reason
that couples who have never been that way shouldn't expect a miraculous transformation just because they are in labour having a baby.

Some childbirth classes and videos create expectations about how
partners *should* behave. They may also feed into a romantic fantasy
where birth inevitably triggers meaningful bonding between the
parents. Disappointment and stress result when couples try to imitate
the videos or rigidly follow a birthing class script. Just be yourselves.

If you anticipate your partner needing more physical or emotional

COUVADE

Couvade, derived from the French word *couver* which means "to hatch, to sit on," is an old custom whereby the father identifies with the labouring mother and participates in bringing their new baby into the world.

When labour begins, the woman stops her daily activities and goes to a birth hut or off into the countryside to give birth by herself. The father, meanwhile, goes to his sleeping area and pretends to be greatly shaken and in need of attention, moaning and groaning until the baby is born.

support than you are capable of giving, don't make yourself or your partner wrong. Give yourself credit for being honest; invite a friend, or hire a doula to be with both of you.

BECOME A GUARDIAN OF THE BIRTH PLACE

Even when a labouring woman is aware of the importance of privacy, warmth, darkness, and quiet, she can't always guard her birth space. If she takes on this role, the resulting anxiety and adrenalin will hinder her progress in labour.

It is difficult to be defensive and trusting at the same time: to be opening to labour while guarding the door. These conflicting tasks create the need for a *guardian of the birth place.*

Many mothers prefer their partners to take the role of birth guardian rather than coach. A birth guardian needs to be calm, sensitive, and sufficiently assertive to handle some of the situations likely to come up.

In the hospital, the guardian's role can

be challenging. Redirecting a flock of medical students, obtaining information about and/or declining optional medical procedures, dimming the lights, and keeping distracting or frightening chatter to a minimum are a few examples.

PROTECT HER PRIVACY

Animals will not labour or birth in an unfamiliar environment, with distracting noise, or in the presence of watchful humans. Like other mammals, human mothers may unconsciously or instinctively inhibit their labour or birth in a situation that feels unfamiliar, if not unsafe.

Having her privacy protected doesn't mean being left alone or abandoned. She needs you there because she feels connected to you and has trust in you.

Think of yourself as a "traffic controller"—restrict well-meaning callers and visitation. Turn off the phone. Close the door. It may help to hang a sign on the door announcing "No Visitors."

THE PAINFUL AFTERMATH OF AN UNGUARDED BIRTH

The following story illustrates how even a supportive father may be overwhelmed by the frenetic unfolding of events in a hospital birth. This is especially likely to happen when he has not had an opportunity in advance to understand how important his role as guardian of the birth place is.

Peggy and Mike planned to birth their first child at home. Upon discovering their baby was breech, their midwife taught Peggy the breech-tilt exercise. When this did not turn their baby around, the midwife referred them to a doctor who attempted to turn the baby by external version. Nevertheless, as their due date approached it was clear that their baby was to be born breech. Arrangements were made for Peggy to birth at a teaching hospital willing to deliver breech babies vaginally. Peggy described what happened next:

> I went into the hospital oriented toward birthing naturally and without drugs. I felt I was doing well with labour, but there was one nurse who was *determined* I should not have *any* pain. In spite of my having declined her offer for drugs, she sent in the doctor with his epidural tray! I couldn't believe it.

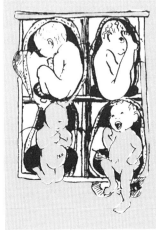

DID YOU KNOW?

Three percent of all babies are breech at term.

In the "four-womb apartment" above, you'll see the four types of breeches: complete, frank, kneeling and footling.

(SEE APPENDIX B FOR
BREECH TILT EXERCISES)

I felt like I had to battle constantly. I had to battle against the epidural, against the clock, against an internal foetal monitor. Going to the bathroom was a hassle—I had to call a nurse every half hour to unhook the monitor and move the machines. Every time someone came in it was a new face.

All through labour there was a tension in the air. I could feel the clock ticking away. I could hear them talking outside my door about "the breech case" and *their* "golden opportunity to see a breech delivery" and so on. I felt like the birth of my child was a clinical-learning circus.

I started to push, they rushed me down the hall to a delivery room. The lights were incredibly bright, they were so bright they seemed blue. Lying on my back I had to look up into them. I felt exposed. The room (temperature) was somewhat cold, and cold in a surgical way. Everyone was in gown and gloves. Sterile sheets covered everything. It gave the room a death-like feeling.

Everyone was in a panic. I felt the urge to push but they didn't want me to push until *they* were ready, until they were gowned, until they were ready to cut the episiotomy.

There were about twenty people in masks and caps in the delivery room. I was flat on my back, my legs were in stirrups, and I felt like the crowd that had gathered was an audience. Five or six (people) were between my legs. Two delivered my baby, one did the episiotomy, another sewed it up, and one was in and out—I don't know what she was doing.

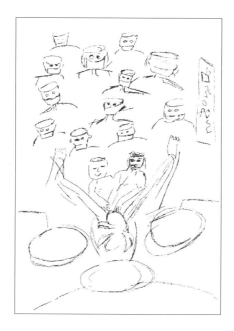

FIGURE 29.1 "This is my strongest image, the most traumatic, troubling image. It shows my sense of having been violated. I've disconnected myself from my body, especially my genitals. I felt incredibly exposed and violated by the hospital birth with 25 spectators and people taking over my body. It was a degrading experience, I felt out of control, at their mercy, objectified, judged and like I had a rare disease having a breech baby, like there was something wrong with me and my baby. I still haven't come to terms with that."

– PEGGY

All this happened even though Mike was nearby providing support. While Peggy did give birth vaginally, little else about the birth was normal. The birth experience and memories were traumatic and plagued her with feelings of anger, violation, and failure. Six months later she came to see me and, through art therapy, began to resolve her grief. When we began I asked her to draw a picture of the birth. She made Figure 29.1 in pencil.

OFFER REALISTIC SUPPORT

A man's lack of experience lessens his credibility when it comes to offering predictions and reassurances about what's unfolding during labour. Often when a father says, "You're doing fine," a woman may snarl (or think to herself) "How the [expletive deleted] would you know?" Yet when her midwife, doula, or mother offers the same encouragement, the labouring woman accepts it.

However, commenting on what you see is a safe bet ("I've never seen you look so strong and determined"); or an expression of tender appreciation ("I love you for bringing our baby into the world"). Women are encouraged when the assurances of a mother, doula, or midwife are repeated, "You're making great progress ... everyone says you're doing fine."

WHAT IF YOUR WIFE "FREAKS OUT?"

One thing you should keep in mind is that almost every woman nearing the end of labour, especially without drugs, *will* become restless, begin looking for a way out (begging for drugs), start doubting herself, and even panic. This sudden and dramatic shift in affect and behaviour is usually brief and occurs just before the urge to push.

Because this is in sharp contrast to the trance-like state of concentration that preceded it, it may be disconcerting and even alarming to a father inexperienced in birth. Realize that this healthy burst of energy is fuelled by a rush of adrenalin, partly due to the building intensity of labour. It's also nature's way of rousing the mother from Labourland's sleepy trance. She needs to be pumped up to push her baby out and to protect it.

When this happens, it is primordial and unconscious. In this state, she is vulnerable to suggestion, so if she sees worry and doubt on your face, she may believe she can't do it and give up. Your eyes should radiate trust, love and confidence. Speak in a calm, reassuring voice; remember she can make it through this last gate of labour.

DON'T BE THE PHOTOGRAPHER

I remember attending a wonderful birth of which the most enduring memory is the father gasping that the camera was out of film—just as the child's head was nearly crowning! While the mother controlled her strong urge to push, the father frantically reloaded the camera.

*

Elli became active, rocking and pacing the floor just before she began pushing. Seeing her in this state, her boyfriend felt a little helpless and anxious. Needing to do *something*, he ran for the video camera and started following Elli around at close range, narrating the labour scene.

Without warning she turned and shouted at him to "GET THAT G*A@Z# THING OUT OF MY FACE!" His eyes widened and he quickly put down the video camera. Later they both experienced regret: she for yelling at him, and he for not having been more sensitive.

A couple needs to decide where the father's focus should be at moments like these. It is disheartening for the mother when her emotional anchor suddenly cuts loose to snap a picture or adjust the video camera, leaving her adrift.

So, if you want your labour and birth in pictures, consider having someone else be your birth photographer.

TAKE CARE OF YOURSELF

Don't expect or wait for *your* needs to be noticed. The father and birth companions often are "invisible." Even during a long labour, no one is likely to offer you a break so you can eat, take a nap or use the bathroom.

If you're birthing in a hospital, consider bringing your own food, or prepare to face food from the cafeteria or vending machines.

Chapter 30

The First Moments

I was at the birth of my two children. I felt them being
born—it was amazing.

STEVIE WONDER

(SIGHTLESS MOTOWN STAR)

SEEING YOUR BABY'S ORIGINAL FACE

It is a rare moment to witness the mystery of birth. if you are distracted by the surge of medical activity (or holding a camera), you
could be right there and miss it! Practise non-focused awareness
(described in Chapter 38) during this transcendent moment:

> See the colour of your baby's wet hair,
> the movement of its head,
> its first expression.
> As its body is being born,
> notice the amniotic fluid pouring
> from its nose and mouth
> (naturally clearing its airway
> for its first breath).
> Watch your baby see for the first time,
> with eyes both empty and full,
> indescribably beautiful.
> Listen to the mother's primal cries of birth …
> and the baby's first cry.
> Feel the baby's warm, wet body, the pulsating cord,
> and the feelings pulsing within you
> as you witness this birth.

*

Babies' reactions to separation from the womb and being born are unknown. But, by imagining what your baby is experiencing you'll be more sensitive in welcoming her to your world. Close your eyes and consider what your baby's life is like in the womb.

Imagine your whole life had been this meditative dream. Then suddenly you are thrust into bright light, cold air, harsh noises, brisk movements, and rough fabric rubbing against your velvet soft skin.

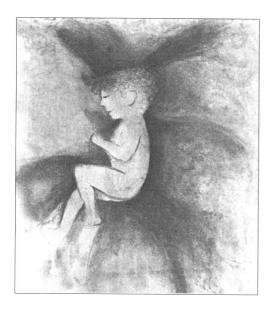

Warmth and darkness,
Floating
Curled up in a soft, snug world.
Silence,
Visited by muted voices and the drumming of mother's heartbeat.
Rhythmic rocking;
Peaceful.."

David's pastel drawing of *A Womb With A View* depicts his baby "cradled in nothing but comfort. Nothing else is important."

Doctors used to hang babies upside down and slap their bottoms (and more recently, flick their feet) to make them cry, believing that intense crying was good for babies because it opened up their lungs. In *Mamatoto: A Celebration of Birth*, we learn that other cultures have similar rituals: "the Abron of the Ivory Coast splash their young with cold water, and in Haiti, a large wooden bowl used to be inverted over the baby and beaten like a drum to wake it up!"[1]

The insensitive obstetric practices described above were challenged by Frederick Leboyer in his book, *Birth Without Violence* (1974). This book, in which he describes his approach in passionate prose accompanied by moving photography, created a stir in the world of obstetrics.

Leboyer, an obstetrician who had delivered 10,000 babies in Paris during his 40 years of practice, believed a baby's intense crying and dramatic body tension at birth are signs of terror, not healthy vigour. In an effort to decrease birth trauma for newborn babies, Leboyer concentrated on making the transition from the womb to the outside world a gentle one. He dimmed lights, quieted voices, and massaged the newborn as it lay on its mother's belly. Sometimes he even murmured chants he'd learned in India.

In an effort to make the first separation from the mother a pleasant one, Leboyer immersed the newborn baby into a warm bath. He wanted to return the baby to the watery environment with which she was familiar. In her Leboyer bath, the baby opens her eyes and looks around; she may smile or seem to fall asleep. Her blue hands and feet turn pink. The bath is not used to wash the baby, it's simply a gentle, sensual welcome to her new world.

Then, as now, some medical professionals argued that the baby could not be properly assessed in dim light, and that a warm bath would chill the baby. But Leboyer, who attended his last 1000 births using this approach (and other birth attendants who've used this approach with thousands of babies), found no adverse effects. However, parents and professionals have observed that babies born into a gentle birth awareness cry less, open their eyes and look around, and have bodies which are noticeably more relaxed.

*

After your baby is born, the cord will continue pulsating for about five minutes, "breathing" oxygen into your baby while she learns to breathe. It's customary for the father to cut the cord, setting the baby free.

THE UNFOLDMENT PROCESS

In order to help awaken the protective parents within, and to create awareness of birth from the *baby's* point of view, our classes offer an elaborate guided visualization which then flows into an experiential exercise called the Unfoldment Process. We want parents to get a feel for how the baby might experience labour contractions; the water breaking; the mother's changing rhythm and sounds; and being pushed into the world.

Before beginning, each couple decides who will play the "uterus/mother," and who will be the "foetus/newborn baby." The "foetus" curls up on the floor in foetal position (what else?!). Then, the "uterus/mother" enfolds the "foetus" in a sheet or blanket. Kneeling close to the "foetus," the "uterus" wraps his/her arms snugly around the baby.

Couples are guided through "labour" in the candle-lit teaching room while soothing music plays. The "contracting uterus" intermittently squeezes the "foetus," contained in its dark, warm, muffled world. On cue, the baby is "born," then has its compressed limbs tenderly unfolded by the "mother." The baby is gently greeted, cradled and rocked in its "mother's" arms.

After the exercise, parents are asked to talk about what labour felt like as a uterus, mother, or baby; and what they learned and want to remember when they welcome their own newborn into the world.

Your baby's newborn assessment (APGAR) can be done on the mother's belly.

Take photographs with fast film (400 ASA or higher) to avoid the disturbance of flash photography.

*

Let the baby adjust to all her new sensations. Take time to see her for the first time, and luxuriate in the miracle that just happened.

There's no need to rush her into nursing. Babies usually are ready to nurse between 20 and 50 minutes after they are born. Wait until your baby crawls up to your nipple or begins rooting before helping her latch on.

Most mothers and babies take their Leboyer bath about an hour after birth. Have someone help you prepare your baby's bath and lay out the baby's outfit, bonnet, socks, receiving blanket and a soft towel. If you are at home or have a tub in your hospital birth room, it's enjoyable to get in the bathtub with your baby.

The room should be warm, but not steamy or hot (which could make you feel faint).

Remember that the baby will be looking up at the ceiling, so turn off the lights. Votive candles around the tub and bathroom are a nice touch.

Get in the tub first (which you will find refreshing after the blood, sweat, and tears of labour). You will probably bleed in the bath water, but this will not affect the baby.

When you're ready, have someone pass your undressed baby to you. Now, holding the baby between your legs, with one hand under her head/neck and the other under her bottom, re-introduce your

---

HOW TO WELCOME YOUR BABY:

- Near the end of labour, warm up the room by turning off the air-conditioner or stoking the fire.
- Dim the lights.
- When the baby is born, be still.
- If you must speak, speak softly.
- Receive your wet, wriggly baby, skin-to-skin.
- Cover your baby with a soft, warm blanket, (At home, during pushing, the blanket can be warmed in a dryer or on a heating pad; in the hospital warm blankets can often be found in a blanket-warmer in the recovery or delivery rooms.)
- Gently, rhythmically stroke your baby's back.
- Softly sing a lullaby or a song to celebrate the birth, or say a prayer.

baby to water by slowly immersing her entire body except for her face. It's okay to get the baby's ears and cord wet.

Most babies like being in the water for about ten minutes.

When her bathtime is up, pass her to someone who will wrap and dry her in the soft towel.

*

If you and your baby are separated or a Leboyer bath is not permitted in your hospital, you can make time later. As soon as you can, hold your baby, and speak to her softly and soothingly. Tell her that the birth was hard or scary, but that it's all right now.

Begin where you are; it's never too late. Put your baby skin-to-skin and nurse her. Even if you have to wait a few days to give the bath (as I did with Sky, who was born by Caesarean), do it when you can.

NURTURING AND CELEBRATING YOUR BABY'S MOTHER

How will you embrace and re-connect with the disheveled, pale and sweaty mother who has just opened wide her body, mind and soul to give birth? She is vulnerable now, tired or weak from the ordeal, and increasingly aware of strangers in the room. She may become self-conscious realizing her genitals are exposed (especially if she's in stirrups), or perhaps she is wondering what people are thinking about how she gave birth ("Did I make too much noise?" "Was I a wimp?").

Too often the baby and the mother's vital signs dominate the foreground of the birth room; no one looks at the mother's face or speaks directly to her for a good while after birth. Nurses bustle about: there's the baby to weigh, notes to make in the chart and a room to clean up. The birth attendant may be busy sewing up an episiotomy. The excited father calls relatives or takes the baby to the nursery—and the mother is left alone.

The mother is reluctant to complain or draw attention to herself because everyone seems to view the new baby as more important.

Birth in our culture is a baby-centred event. But babies usually need very little at birth. They enjoy nestling against the mother's warm body under a soft blanket, or nuzzling new-found breasts—in harmony with what the mother is able to give.

More often than not, a woman who's just given birth needs a few minutes to "get back in her body" as she returns from the intensity of hormonal Labourland. Only then can she give full attention to the baby.

A mother exhausted or devastated after a particularly difficult labour may not be interested in looking at or holding her baby for a few minutes, and sometimes longer. If her wishes are respected, without pressuring her or inducing guilt, this well-deserved recuperation time will help her begin mothering on a positive note. When the mother is ready, the two of you can discover the baby together.

So, fathers or birth companions, after the baby is born, wrap your love around the mother. Tell her softly how much you love and appreciate what she gave to bring the baby into the world.

Often, women shake involuntarily, sometimes violently, right before and after birthing. A Native-American mother told me that they attribute the shaking to the Soul entering the baby's body.

If your partner is shaking from head to toe, instead of telling her to relax to stop the shaking, suggest she "relax into the shaking" and reassure her it will stop in a little while. Labour-shivers feel better when being held in strong arms and a warm blanket. If

"I complained. I wanted the miserable labouring to end. In the midst of it all, however, I knew something cataclysmic was happening to me. In my struggle to open myself and let the baby be born, something else was opening as well—some aperture between me and what was beyond me. Swept through this opening as if by a tidal bore, my senses were overwhelmed by a rushing, roaring momentum driving me to the margins of not only what I could bear but what I could comprehend.

The my baby arrived, slithering out into waiting hands, joining our human circle and completing it. At that moment, the wormhole to infinity snapped shut. I was cut off forever from some magnificent mystery. I was beached, quivering and raw, on the sands of everyday life."

– CHRISTINE HALE
"BIRTH AT HOME: AN IMMANENT POWER"[2]

she is cold, put socks on her feet. Another kind gesture is to bring the new mother cold juice to raise her blood sugar and moisten her dry mouth. If you are snuggled up with her, send someone else for it.

*

OFF TO THE NURSERY

At home, the baby is never separated from the mother or father immediately after birth. The newborn examination is done on the bed with the parents participating.

If you are birthing in the hospital, policies vary widely; learn what to expect beforehand. Some hospitals may perform the examination in the birth room, but most still insist that the baby be taken to the nursery for about three hours for an examination, bath and rewarming.

Even if the policy at your hospital is to send healthy babies to the nursery soon after birth, you can request an exception to the rule. If your hospital won't cooperate and you must take the baby to the nursery, here are some things to keep in mind:

MOTHER ROASTING

Many cultures have postpartum customs of "roasting, baking, steaming, or poaching" the cold, shaking, weak new mother. They believe heat shrinks the uterus, restores strength and stimulates production of milk.

Around the world, mothers are warmed:

soaking in steaming baths,
with hot rocks
wrapped in cloths,
by crackling fires,
swaddled in toasty blankets
heated in stoves or dryers,
by turning up the thermostat
in a chilly hospital,
and even squatting over ashes taken from a sacred fire.

Most mothers are not ready to be separated (they've waited so long for this moment). A routine nursery policy of this kind obviously violates all natural instincts. Even if it's unspoken, be aware of the mother's possible disappointment, and soften the separation by acknowledging her loss (and not gloating over your good fortune).

Within an hour or two of giving birth—of experiencing one of the most amazing, intense, life-changing events in her life—a mother is left alone to wait (usually two to three hours or even more) for the father and baby to return from the nursery. During this tender time, a mother needs to be mothered, helped with a bath or shower, have her hair brushed, and given a nutritious meal; she needs to talk about the birth. Being left alone during this time is lonely, anticlimactic, and even cruel. Here's where the continuous support of a woman friend, relative or doula makes a huge difference!

*

Fathers, stay with your baby in the nursery and participate in the exam. Your baby will be given eye ointment to prevent infection that could lead to blindness, and a vitamin K shot to protect against a rare, but serious, bleeding condition. You can ask your paediatrician or nurse for more information on these standard procedures.

TREE OF LIFE

In many cultures it's a custom to plant a fruit tree in honour of a new baby. To celebrate your baby's birth, consider giving the placenta back to the earth to nourish the roots of a tree. As your baby grows, its tree will grow, too.

One day, when Luc was four years old, he was watering his placenta-cherry tree. He looked up at me and said proudly, "Mummy, my placenta is really special! It grew me *and* my cherry tree."

Nurseries routinely give the baby a bath. These days, the bath helps protect hospital staff from contracting HIV or Hepatitis B, which can be passed from an infected baby's (unwashed) skin. If your baby doesn't get a bath, the nurses will wear gloves when caring for it.

There is no other reason to bathe a baby soon after birth. In fact, there are some disadvantages. If the bath is given quickly under running water in the sink, it can be frightening and upsetting to the newborn. A baby's temperature drops after this ordeal, so, to prevent a complication called "cold stress," your baby must be re-warmed. Rather than warming the baby by skin-to-skin cuddling with the mother, most nurseries put the baby under "warming lights" in the nursery for three hours. The time your baby's gone may not be significant when compared to a life-time, but it *feels* like forever to a mother who is waiting.

Remember, you, as the father, can decline the routine baby bath. Midwives at one hospital told me they encourage every couple to write to the administrator about any grievances concerning outdated policies requiring separation of a healthy mother and baby. It is consumers who change bureaucratic or obsolete regulations.

Chapter 31

Labourland Etiquette

Labourland is in some ways a fragile state. When you enter the labour room, bring with you an attitude of gentleness, respect, even reverence. The mother's chance of progressing well during labour improves when rules and customs that preserve the body-mind harmony of labour are observed. Here are some things to be aware of:

REMEMBER THE IMPORTANCE OF PRIVACY

Birth isn't a "happening" or a party. It's almost as private as lovemaking. The celebration can begin *after* the mother has given birth. To protect privacy, you're going to need a "traffic controller."

CHOOSE YOUR TRAFFIC CONTROLLER BEFORE LABOUR BEGINS

Two potentially tricky questions you face are:

- 1. Who should be at the birth?
- 2. Which person will have the responsibility to manage visitation for the mother's best interest?

Because the first question involves making choices, compromises, and perhaps even painful boundary setting, there may be a temptation to avoid it entirely. Sometimes a friend or relative assumes that, of course, she/he will be at the birth with you. This becomes awkward if you don't want that person, or additional people, there during your private experience. You'll have to decide whether having your birth place be the way you want it is worth the risk of hurt feelings or conflict resulting from drawing necessary boundaries.

As for the second question, choose someone (perhaps the father or doula) who can be sensitive, tactful, gracious, and when necessary, firm. Make sure this person knows how to read the mother's cues during labour about whom she's wanting to be present.

SPEAK LABOURLAND'S NATIVE TONGUE

When labour begins, most women are talkative, sociable and hyper-alert. The burst of energy that accompanies the onset of labour allows for last minute "nesting." Both of you can use this opportunity to take care of any unfinished business before settling into your birth place.

As labour progresses, chemical-hormonal changes in the brain bring about a quiet, internally-focused state of mind. Eventually, interest in her labour-project will wane. She will become indifferent or annoyed by chit-chat, and the s p a c e s b e t w e e n h e r t h o u g h t s a n d w o r d s w i l l w i d e n. Except when interrupted by contractions, she may appear to be in a trance, if not "asleep." She is now in Labourland.

With few exceptions, the further along in labour a woman is, the more difficult it becomes for her to ask or answer questions, make decisions, or even respond with a simple "yes" or "no." This is a positive sign that she has shifted from her left-brain to her right-brain (her primitive birthing-brain).

It is only after her logical, rational, verbal left-brain comes to a screaming halt, that her intuitive, unconscious right-brain takes over to carry her through a journey that can't be navigated intellectually.

This shift from left- to right-brain, from conscious to unconscious, facilitates the surrender required in active labour. Without that shift, wherein mind and ego melt into the background, most women could not stand the intensity of active labour.

You, and everyone in attendance, should respectfully encourage this mysterious phenomenon. It helps if you are fluent in the language of Labourland. Speak softly, slowly, using simple phrases to avoid disrupting her labour-trance or concentration.

QUIET! BIRTHING ZONE

A mother's introspective state and sudden lack of communication leaves fathers feeling lonely and disconnected. Some fathers try to reconnect through talking; ask yourself whose needs this will meet.

If other people are engaging in chit-chat, talking technology, expressing fears, telling scary birth stories or asking endless questions—the mother will be drawn out of labour's perfect trance (right-brain) and into her intellect (left-brain). This shift makes her coping with labour more difficult, and can cause labour to slow down, or even stop.

Respectful silence from those in attendance is especially important during contractions (they require intense concentration). Unless you are talking her through the contraction, don't talk to her, or to others (whispering is especially aggravating to a labouring woman).

OFFER—DON'T ASK

A woman's ability to verbalize her needs in active labour is usually impaired by the normal neuro-hormonal changes in the brain. Certain women may be further impaired by upbringings which discouraged asking for what they need, or saying no when they don't want something.

Therefore, try to anticipate the mother's unspoken needs. For example, a woman in labour needs to drink about a quarter of a pint of fluid per hour. From time to time, offer the glass or straw by putting it up to her mouth. If she is thirsty, she will drink. If not, she will turn her head, or even swat at the glass (don't take it personally!).

Also, try to avoid complex questions like: "Do you want apple juice, cranberry juice, or ice chips?" … Too many choices. Pick *one* and offer it.

> Only offer a labouring woman three fingers to squeeze in labour … she is apt to break a finger if she squeezes all four at once.

LET HER FINGERS DO THE TALKING

This is helpful in situations where it's hard to guess what the mother wants. "At one point," Analisa recalled, "there were five close friends in my labour room but I just wanted us to be alone. I was so relieved when my husband, Romaldo, said, 'There are a lot of people in here.

Do you want me to ask them to leave for a while?' I raised one of my fingers, a signal we had agreed upon before labour, and he knew what I wanted."

BEWARE OF: RELAX! OR BREATHE!

What does saying "relax" to a woman in active labour mean anyway? Real labour is no time to relax completely, it's time to *work hard*. It's okay for a woman to rock on her hands and knees during a painful contraction, or squeeze a pillow or your hand if that helps. Being active and strong is part of coping with the pain and getting the baby out.

The futility of trying to relax completely in labour causes some women to become discouraged when they can't reach the deep state of relaxation they achieved in class. If labour is long or difficult, they may think it is because they did not relax well enough. Such self-criticism only adds to their tension.

So, if you really want to help her, don't keep telling her to "Relax!" If she could relax, she would. Nobody would like to "relax" more than she, but she can't until the baby is born!

If you can't think of what else to say, try acknowledging how strong she is or how well she is working with the pain and exhaustion. Incorporate suggestions that evoke images of relaxation such as:

- As you breathe out … your ligaments (cervix, bones) are beginning to soften (stretch, release)
- Feel your (pelvis, cervix, thighs) soften (yield, release, open) with each contraction … a little bit more … with each breath out
- Expand, unfold, trust …
- Keep faith, believe in …
- The pain is strong, but you are stronger than the pain …
- You are bringing our baby soon …

*

The same holds true for "Breathe … Breathe!," or insisting she follow a specific breathing pattern taught in class. Most midwives I know scoff at labour breathing "techniques" because they know they can undermine a woman's natural adaptation to labour. In nature, mothers instinctively arrive at a breathing pattern which matches their labour. Even if she's learned particular breathing techniques, the mother will discover her own unique rhythm or pattern in labour.

IT'S A LABOUR ROOM (NOT A DINING ROOM)

In order to keep up their strength, mothers can and should eat during early labour. However, during active labour, the sight and smell of food usually is aversive, even sickening, to them.

But there's no reason for *you* not to eat. So don't feel guilty if you're hungry and want to take a break to eat. Just don't eat in the labour room. Afterwards, brush your teeth or rinse your mouth so the smell of food doesn't upset her stomach.

EXIT GRACEFULLY

When you need to take a break, don't announce, "I'm LEAVING you …" A labouring woman's grip becomes amazingly strong upon hearing these words, making it nearly impossible for you to leave. It's better to say, "I'll be right back, I need to take a little break," and return as quickly as you can. Having a doula or woman friend in the room makes it possible for you to take guilt-free father-breaks.

KEEP YOUR REMINDER CARDS HANDY

I give fathers and birth companions three pocket-card reminders*: the first summarizes labour support suggestions, the second is a list of pain-coping techniques learned in class, and the third (found in the next chapter) contains guidelines for gathering information in order to give informed consent and make better decisions about your medical care. I encourage people to bring these cards to their births.

*Permission is granted for reproduction by parents reading this book for personal use. To reproduce for publication or education, obtain permission in writing from authors.

HELPFUL REMINDERS FOR FATHERS AND OTHER BIRTH COMPANIONS

REMEMBER THE IMPORTANCE OF:

- Protect privacy, turn off the phone, close the door, restrict visitors. Birth is not a happening/She is not a party hostess.
- Observe/anticipate her needs. Don't ask too many questions.
- Respectful silence, or talk to her slowly, softly during contractions.
- Use non-verbal signals.
- Suggest bath or shower, change in position, walking, voiding.
- Encourage sips of a nutritive drink, at least a quarter of a pint an hour. Choose sports drinks, tea with honey, juice (not just water/ice chips).
- Wear the hide of an encyclopedia salesman—don't take any rejection or reaction personally.

PAIN-COPING TECHNIQUES

REMEMBER:

- Be curious about the pain
- Notice what's already working … and do more of that
- Breath Awareness
- Build a Partnership With Your Baby
- Non-Focused Awareness (mindful awareness without judging)
- Quaker Listening
- Edges of Sensation
- Edges of Comfort (Where exactly does the sensation begin and end? How does it move/change with each breath out?)
- Centre of Sensation (emptiness/stillness in the eye of the hurricane)
- Spiralling (out of the centre of sensation, moving the spiral with each exhalation)
- Touch Awareness (downward stroke on her outward breath)
- Massage
- Primordial Vocalization or Co-chanting.

Chapter 32

Gathering Information: Guidelines for Making Decisions and Giving Informed Consent

> I wish I had known how to ask the right questions. If I had asked more questions things might have turned out better. I guess I thought that what they were suggesting was the only way to go.
>
> STEVE, A NEW FATHER

Couples accustomed to joint decision-making need to change their style in active labour. In Labourland, a woman's logical and verbal abilities are significantly impaired. Even if she has a question or understands what's being said or asked, she can't always speak up.

In modern, medicalized labour, even during a normal labour, couples often are bombarded with directives and decisions. One of your most difficult tasks is to differentiate between what is routine, optional, and/or necessary.

To a large extent, extracting key information in a given situation falls to the father or birth companion. (That's why we have included this chapter in the Fathers and Birth Companions section.) This is for a number of reasons. First, there is the trance-like nature of labour itself. Then there is women's socialization to be polite and cooperative with authorities. Finally, the psychological vulnerability and dependency accompanying the role of hospital patient can block even the most assertive and educated woman from taking charge.

Some fathers or birth companions may need to be more assertive than they usually would be. She's depending on you, so if questioning or standing up to medical personnel is too uncomfortable for you, be honest with yourself. If you can't do it, have someone at the birth who can.

*

You have the right to receive balanced information before making any decision about your health care. Take responsibility: learn all the facts and alternatives. Then your "yes," or "no," will be a genuine informed decision.

Many parents have found the following questions useful in arriving at an informed decision. The questions are not intended to create confrontation or to communicate mistrust in your birth attendant. Give your birth attendants' intentions the benefit of the doubt.

QUESTIONS TO HELP YOU GET INFORMATION*

TESTS AND PROCEDURES:

- What will we find out from this test/procedure?
- How accurate is it?
- What are the risks?
- Do they outweigh the benefits?
- What will you or we do differently based on the results?
- If nothing, is there another reason to do it?

TREATMENTS, DRUGS AND INTERVENTIONS:

- How will this be helpful?
- Why must this be done now? What might happen if we wait an hour? A week? Or do nothing?
- What are the advantages/disadvantages?
- This may be the treatment you usually recommend but what other approaches can you tell us about?
- If several treatment choices are possible: Is there a logical sequence in which to try the different options?

*This pocket-reminder card is intended for private use by parents, who can cut out the card in Appendix D. Permission to reproduce this card for publication or education must be obtained in writing from authors.

In the Birthing From Within childbirth classes, couples use role plays to practise the questions below. Not only is this entertaining and fun, but fathers get a taste of what it takes to discuss and negotiate birth decisions with medical personnel.

These questions are not just for labour. Use them during prenatal care, or any other health care situation. Keep a copy in your wallet.

*

If you are still undecided, it is your right and responsibility to get a second opinion.

Circumcision

FORESKIN FORETHOUGHT: INFORMED CONSENT

Baby boys depend on their parents to gather and weigh information about circumcision, *before* allowing it to happen. Many parents don't realize that circumcision is not routine or medically necessary, and that they can decline this surgery for their sons.

HOW IS NEWBORN CIRCUMCISION HELPFUL?

In 1971 the American College of Pediatrics stated "There is no valid medical indication for circumcision in the newborn." Seven years later, the American College of Obstetricians and Gynecologists also took a stand against routine circumcision. The procedure has become increasingly unpopular in the US, and in the UK circumcision is generally only carried out for emergency medical conditions.

WHAT ARE THE RISKS?

Haemorrhage, infection, gangrene, septicemia, ulceration of the exposed urinary meatus (from wet diapers), and even loss of the penis. When too much foreskin is removed, skin grafting may need to be done later, resulting in other possible complications. In addition, the penis may become permanently crooked or disfigured.

CIRCUMCISION ENVY?

One morning, when Luc was four, he and I (R.H.) stumbled into the bathroom together. As we competed in our "productivity" contest, Luc noticed our different appearances for the first time.

"Yours looks like a mushroom!," he declared."How come?"

I laughed, and explained that most men my age had had the tip of their penis skin cut off when they were babies, but that Mommy and I hadn't let that be done to him. His brow furrowed with concern as he asked, "Did it hurt you Daddy?" After I answered, he said, "Thank you for not letting them do that to me."

Now, when I see his uncircumcised penis, with its different appearance from mine, I feel a quiet satisfaction that I helped protect his little body from that needless and painful procedure.

A NURSE'S VIEW

I'm an R.N. who has worked for one-and-a-half years in a new-born nursery in a hospital ... When I have to set up a baby for circumcision, I feel like crying and often do. I feel like I'm betraying that being behind those eyes, as I calmly and easily strap him on the "circboard." I talk to him about what will be happening and apologize. After witnessing many circumcisions, I can say: "Yes, it hurts. It's pure and simple torture." As often as I can I leave the room ...

I've talked to parents many times about their babies' circumcision before it's been done. I see fathers just sort of shrug like ... it's one of those things boys have to go through. And mothers who wince at the thought, and hope not to hear his screams, still sign the papers of permission. Parents ask, "Does it hurt him?" and I tell them yes ... But they always have a good reason to go ahead ... "He would be teased." "He wouldn't match his dad (or brothers)." "We've always done it in our family." "It's so much worse if it would have to be done later."

–TERRY SHULTZ, R.N.
FROM A LETTER TO *MOTHERING*

For more on circumcision see Appendix E.

Birthing Through Pain

The Pain and Power of Birth

INTRODUCTION

If you turned to this section first, you are probably wondering what the pain of labour will be like, how best to handle it and if there's a way you can "beat" it. Here's some good news for pain worriers.

Women who worry "the right amount" do the *best* in labour. Why? Because worrying activates searching for resources, both inner and outer. Worrying also motivates you to practice pain-coping techniques while there's still time to master them. On the other hand, women who are over-confident about handling labour pain are in for a surprise.

Some women don't worry about pain because they are planning to use drugs or an epidural during labour. Regardless of your plans, the unexpected can happen, and you should be prepared for it. Sometimes the anaesthesiologist is not immediately available; or labour progresses so quickly that even if you were planning on an epidural, there isn't time for one. Either way you won't regret having learned ways to cope with pain.

*

There are three things Birthing From Within emphasizes:

First, mothers need to learn the difference between feeling pain, and *suffering*. The pain-coping techniques described in this book are intended to help eliminate needless physical and emotional suffering that might otherwise be experienced during labour.

Second, it takes practise to master these techniques. To have brief instruction in pain techniques and then expect to use them to help you manage the most intense pain of your life is much like taking a few skiing classes and thinking you'll be able to handle rocketing down a steep mountain's most difficult run.

It's important to realize that the pain and stress of normal labour are part of what keeps this natural process on track. Here's why you should think twice before trying to *eliminate* pain:

1. The stress hormones produced in response to labour pain help protect your baby against hypoxia (insufficient oxygen) during labour, as well as preparing its lungs for breathing after it is born.
2. "Pain guides the mother. Commonly, the positions and activities she chooses for comfort are also those that promote good labour progress or help shift the baby into the right position for birth. Remove the pain, and you kill that feedback mechanism."[1]
3. Removing pain also severs other feedback loops vital to normal labour and birth. "Nerves in the cervix, and later the pelvic floor muscles and vagina, transmit stretching sensations as well as pain. These stretch receptors signal the pituitary to produce more oxytocin, which increases the tempo of the labour, causing further cervical dilation ... and the urge to push ... Numb the nerves with an epidural, and you also wipe out the positive feedback mechanism."[2]

There are no guarantees how well any of these techniques will work for you in labour. But practising them in your every day life beforehand builds a mindset, a way of being aware and focused. After a while, this skill will become natural for you; in labour you'll just do more of it, with greater concentration (and motivation).

Practising pain-coping techniques also creates an empowering ritual of preparation which is absorbed by your subconscious. So, when your conscious mind is swept away by the intensity and exhaustion of labour, your subconscious resources will be there for you.

Finally, the intensity of labour pain is such that no technique can fulfill a promise of pain-free labour. In fact, the Birthing From Within approach does not advocate birthing without drugs *regardless* of what's happening (See Chapter 39: Compassionate Use of Drugs And Epidurals).

*

Section VI, The Pain and Power of Birth, presents, from three perspectives, things you can do to cope with pain in labour:

- Learning how your attitudes and beliefs influence the extent of suffering in labour.
- Mobilizing environmental and emotional support to make birth easier.
- Practising pain-coping techniques.

*

- And there's a fourth perspective, spirituality, which is vitally important to many people. Spirituality is an essential part of birth preparation. You can bring a picture, statue, prayer, music, or anything else to your birth space that might have spiritual meaning for you. When you are afraid or tired in labour, connecting with your spirituality can be grounding and strengthening.

Chapter 33

Looking For A Way Out

It s difficult enough to be fully "present" when you are comfortable. So, when you're in the midst of pain, or even anticipating it, it's not surprising that you might begin looking for a way out, for something or someone to help you escape.

Many childbirth teachers and health professionals unwittingly have misguided mothers by reinforcing the hope that pain can be avoided, and by supporting our natural childlike tendency to look *outward* for comfort and relief. Turning to drugs or technology to solve problems has become a cultural reflex. Nevertheless, adopting a passive stance to dealing with pain has consequences. Is the reassuring option of analgesics or an epidural keeping you from plumbing the depth of your own resources?

There's a big difference between the mental focus and motivation of a circus tightrope walker who works over a net and one who doesn't. In the same way, if you are planning a hospital birth, the availability of a drug back-up net may undermine the total commitment and concentration necessary to move through your pain. If you want to give birth without drugs, you will need the life-and-death mindfulness of the tightrope artist who works without a net.

Another risk conveyed by the idea that pain can be avoided is that it narrows a woman's vision of how she *should* be controlling labour pain.

One mother confided bitterly to me that in her fear of losing control in labour, she had bought "hook, line, and sinker" the notion that being controlled and relaxed was the right way to give birth. "When I began moaning and rocking and hit the white-knuckle part of labour, I felt I was failing."

Like many mothers nearing the end of labour, this mother was unable to completely relax her arms and hands and breathe quietly through contractions. It became a *problem* because, in the midst of labour, she was unprepared to envision any other coping behaviour. As a result, she resorted to drugs to achieve her only acceptable image of labouring: that of being controlled and quiet.

There are lots of options available, but if you are to give birth instinctively, spontaneously and drug-free, there is virtually nowhere to go but *through* your pain.

GOING A LITTLE DEEPER

It's natural to seek pleasure and avoid pain. It is essential to survival to avoid or fix pain that is life-threatening. But normal labour pain doesn't need to be fixed; it is a healthy sensation that signals your baby is coming, and helps it arrive.

Even so, women today don't have to feel pain to give birth. It is a choice. But, before you make a choice out of fear, consider exploring your assumptions about pain. Anything you "know" that isn't actually happening in the moment is based on assumptions!

Doing the exercises in the following chapters with your birth companion or other couples in childbirth class may help you challenge assumptions and discover new ways of coping with labour pain.

Chapter 34

Exploring Beliefs and Attitudes About Pain

If you haven't explored your personal attitudes and beliefs about pain, learning specific pain techniques is premature, if not pointless. The following five exercises were developed to help you do just that.

I: EXPANDING YOUR PAIN TOLERANCE

Lyn vividly recalls a session with the psychologist she was consulting about her traumatic first birth. He asked her about her expectations for her upcoming (second) labour. Lyn was totally confident this birth would be easier because it was her second. She adamantly dismissed the possibility that her second labour could be as intense or painful as her first. Lyn's fears were rationalized and safely tucked away. Unfortunately, avoidance doesn't get us ready for what awaits us in labour.

Lyn's psychologist challenged her, "But what if it *is* as bad, or worse this time?"

"Oh, it couldn't be! It just couldn't be," Lyn said with a nervous laugh.

"Well, let's just pretend it is twice as long and hard as the first time, what would you do then? You have to do something, what will you do?"

Lyn was unnerved by this line of questioning, yet it compelled her to look more deeply into her fear. This shift led her to begin mobilizing her resources, both internal and external, and she realized she *would* survive another long, hard labour.

While Lyn's second labour was much faster, it was just as painful as her first. She was not taken by surprise or unprepared because she had steeled herself to expect even more pain for this birth.

TRY THIS: "SCALING" PAIN

On a scale of 0–100, with zero being no pain and 100 being the most intense pain you can possibly imagine, rate the expected intensity of your labour pain in:

0 _____ 100
Early labour

0 _____ 100
Middle of labour

0 _____ 100
Completely dilated

1. If the pain is twice as strong as you're expecting, how will you respond? What might be most helpful? Least helpful?
2. Would you like to be alone? Held? Talked through it?

II: YOUR "IDEAL" RESPONSE TO LABOUR PAIN

Describe or draw your image in your journal or talk it over with a friend.

1. Gently explore your image:
   In your ideal image of coping with pain, describe
   what you are doing …
   how you are feeling …
   what you are needing from others …
   and what is most helpful.
2. Investigate ideas: If you think, "I want to be brave, or strong," ask yourself "what does brave or strong mean to me?"
   Investigate how you are brave or strong in your daily life?
3. Help from a support person: If you envision a particular person helping you in labour, ask yourself:

- How does that person help me now?
- Do I *allow* that person to help me now?
- Can I be completely un-self-conscious in labour with that person no matter how I act or what happens?
- What nagging doubts do I have about this person?

III: UNDECIDED ABOUT USING DRUGS?

Exploring the following two scenarios might help. Picture yourself trapped in a cabin in a Montana snow storm. Your labour is in high gear and there are no drugs to be had.

- What do you see yourself doing to cope with the pain?
- What fantasies do you have of other kinds of help that might be available?

*

Suppose you are in a hospital next door to a well-stocked pharmacy. You can have anything you want, whenever you want it, and are encouraged to place an order.

- How will you know when to place the order?
- Besides taking away the pain, how do you imagine drugs helping?

OVERCOMIING PAIN SHAME

- What responses to pain in labour do you consider unacceptable?
- How are those responses a problem for you?
- To whom else would they be unacceptable?
- What would those responses mean about you?
- What would you say to another woman who coped with her pain in those ways?

IV: ASHAMED OF USING DRUGS IN LABOUR?

If you want/need drugs but think you would be a failure for using them, ask yourself:

- How might drugs be helpful to you in labour?
- What do you believe about women who use drugs in labour?
- Is your belief influenced by somebody who's important to you?
- What is it you might regret if you use drugs or an epidural during labour?
- What concerns do you have about the effects of analgesics or epidural on your baby?

Chapter 35

Endorphins

How have women historically survived the pain of childbirth without drugs? They had no choice, but luckily, nature prepared women's bodies for such an event.

When the brain perceives pain (especially with the added stimulus of stress) endorphins are released. Endorphins are chemical compounds secreted by the brain and adrenal glands, and have a pain-relieving effect ten times more potent than morphine. They also are mood elevators (e.g., "runner's high").

As dilation progresses the sensation of pain will increase. The more pain you have, the more endorphins are released to help you cope. The rising level of endorphins contributes to the shift from a thinking, rational mindset to a more primitive and instinctive one. Endorphins take you to the dream-like state of Labourland, which meshes well with the tasks of birthing.

A SOFTER MEMORY OF BIRTH

Endorphins also can have a dramatic impact on how we remember our births. Having given birth with and without drugs, I was fascinated by how drugs affected my memory:

> Late into my first labour, I was given an epidural in preparation for my Caesarean. The endorphin haze lifted suddenly, much as if a curtain had been raised. I became absolutely aware of my surroundings; everything around me was in sharp focus again. My memories are still distinct: the clock on the wall, time passing, sterile blue drapes, glaring lights, medical conversation and the clanging of instruments. Years later my fear and loneliness associated with those moments remain vivid.

Without the endorphin haze, memories are shaped and stored in a way that makes them more vivid when retrieved. After an epidural, *external* events seize the foreground of awareness (and later, memory), displacing the softer inner experience and emotions which ordinarily would be part of protecting against lasting trauma.

I realized talking to Rob one day that it was nature's intent, through endorphins, to keep us "out of our mind" in labour. With this come additional gifts: amnesia about the pain and a misty magical memory. I wonder if part of the trauma of Caesarean or difficult births, in which medication is used, is that women's memories of them are painfully acute.

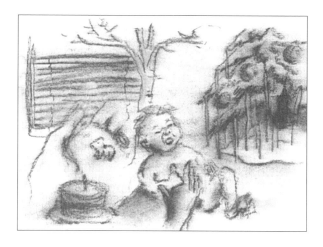

My memory of my second birth, in which I had no drugs, is more like viewing an impressionist painting through a veil. Not only was the birth gentler and kinder in every way, but so are my memories of it.

Chapter 36

The Ecology of Pain

Pain is *experienced* in the brain, yet is shaped by a tremendous range of external factors. The response to pain is partially determined by its ecology, i.e., the physical and social environment. Your birth place, and the people in it, play a vital role in your relationship with pain.

THE TERRAIN OF PAIN IS MAINLY IN THE BRAIN

HOW CAN MY BIRTH PLACE HELP ME COPE WITH PAIN?

To understand the way birth environment influences our responses in birth, some background in brain development may be helpful. The primitive part of our brain (the brain stem) is the part we have in common with other mammals. Our primitive brain controls instinctive behaviour and regulates automatic responses of organs and systems.

Through evolution, the capacity for language and thought developed, and was localized in the "new" brain (which covers the primitive brain). The new brain (with its propensity to Think) can inhibit instinctive, primal activities such as sex and birth. Clinical/cognitive birth environments engage the new brain with their demands for complex decision-making.

On the other hand, there are birth environments which tend to connect more readily with the primitive brain processes at the core of giving birth. Those birth environments are characterized by: privacy, warmth and darkness, water, freedom of movement and an equal relationship with the people attending the birth. Let's consider how each of these areas affects your experience of pain:

PRIVACY AND SUPPORT

People who are at your birth should be people with whom you feel connected and who have trust in you. They can help you feel less self-conscious and more relaxed and secure, all of which can help you cope with pain. On the other hand, too many people, or the wrong people, can heighten anxiety, self-consciousness, and increase your experience of pain.

WARMTH AND DARKNESS

Although a brightly-lit labour room may be helpful for clinicians, such an environment can intensify pain, feelings of being exposed or watched, and raise performance anxiety in a labouring mother. While bright lights or a cool room inhibit relaxation and stimulate the release of adrenalin, a warm, dimly-lit room generates relaxation and peace of mind in the labouring mother. I have often seen mothers gravitate toward a quiet back room, and draw the shades. Being wrapped in a warm blanket, or massaged with hot oil during a long and tiring labour can restore a feeling of well-being. This physical and psychological comfort reduces adrenalin, thereby facilitating the effectiveness of the birth-enhancing hormone, oxytocin.

WATER

Water has its unique way of helping in labour. Water bubbling in a brook, waves washing ashore, the trickle of a garden fountain all inspire relaxation. In labour, sometimes just the sound of running water can help move things along.

When you are restless during *active* labour (6 cm or more), or if you are dilating slowly, soaking in a warm bath eases pain as well as decreases adrenalin. It is not unusual for a woman to dilate much more quickly in a warm bath or shower.

"In the highlands of New Guinea, a Gahuku woman gives birth by the riverside, where she can watch the dark green of the water lapping up against the banks while other women bathe her back and shoulders with cloths dipped in the river."[2]

In her article, "Therapeutic Effects of Bathing During Labour," Christine Brown explains how the uterus and surrounding abdominal muscles are acutely sensitive to pressure during labour. If a woman tenses her abdominal muscles during a contraction, the pain of the contraction will increase. A mother immersed in warm water experiences a feeling of weightlessness, deeper abdominal muscle relaxation, and therefore less pain. The uterus is able to contract more efficiently.[1]

In early or latent labour, a warm lavender bath may help a mother relax and progress in labour. If labour stops or slows down after the excitment of being admitted to a hospital, a warm, soothing bath may get labour started again. However, be aware that taking long, *hot baths* does not always have the same helpful effect during normal early labour (in fact, it can slow it down).

Brown notes that "the optimum temperature for the relief of pain is about that of blood and deeper body tissues. If you are taking a bath, the temperature should be comfortably warm, 98–100°F." When the bath water cools, add more hot water. If the bath is too warm, or you stay in too long, you may actually lose energy and become tired and weak. A cold washcloth on your forehead and chest, drinking cold juice, and getting out of the water to cool off periodically, all help avoid overheating.

Studies show that being in a bath during active labour does not increase the risk of infection (even when the water has broken).[3]

MUSIC

In labour, women naturally focus on sounds around them. If you can, take a walk outside. Listening to birds, the wind or rain is soothing. Once you're confined inside, have a variety of music on hand.

> People never sing ... except in the bathroom. Birthing women also make their natural sounds next to running bath water. There is something aboiut the power of water. People are drawn to water, spas, and sacred streams. Women in labour are drawn to water, too."
>
> – MICHEL ODENT, MD

If labour is intense and you can't relax, listening to soothing music, the sounds of whales, or other sounds from nature can be helpful.

On the other hand, if labour is slow, or you're tired and need to re-energize, music that makes you want to move is what you're after.

FREEDOM OF MOVEMENT

I've yet to hear a woman tell me that lying still in labour eased her pain. The rituals (routines) of putting on a hospital gown, lying down, signing permits for treatment, anaesthesia, being hooked up to a monitor and an IV, all move a woman from a position of action and independence to one of dependence and passivity.

These widely-practiced birth rituals subtly inform the mother that to be a responsible mother she must be a "good" patient. This done, not only is a woman's physical movement restricted, but her psychological freedom, intuition and assertion are diminished as well. In a sense, these are rites of regression rather than rites of empowerment.

In contrast, a woman up and about in her birth room, or one tending to her garden or dishes, is perceived as a strong, healthy woman just having a baby. An environment in which a woman can be physically active and engaged in normal activities also allows her to discover the most comfortable and effective physical positions.

AROMATHERAPY

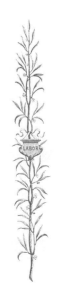

Whether you are birthing at home or in the hospital, the fragrance from oils extracted from flowers, plants, trees, fruit, and roots can calm and comfort the body-mind in pregnancy and labour. Doulas often bring aromatherapy oils to labour to replace clinical odors in the hospital that may unconsciously affect the mother's body-mind in labour.

In her article, "Aromatherapy for Childbearing," Marlene Ericksen recommends the following:

Pregnancy Perineal Massage Blend of 3 drops of lavender, 1 drop of geranium and I ounce of wheat germ oil. Neroli, bergamot, rose, and frankincense can help relieve anxiety and fears.

Lavender can promote relaxation and pain relief. Let the aroma of one drop of oil permeate the room, or take a 30 minute lavender bath in early labour. Some women like a lavender foot massage.

To help stimulate and strengthen contractions, try a jasmine (*Jasminum grandiflorum*) compress on the lower abdomen or sacrum.[4]

SOCIAL MESSAGES ABOUT HOW TO COPE WITH PAIN

Our culture is relearning, painfully, that a birth environment is much more than the stage on which technology performs. In fact your birth place often dictates the script that will be played out.

The attitude and behaviour of hospital staff are affected by the environmental design of the birth place. If labour rooms are closely spaced or shared by other labouring women, nurses may be more inclined to encourage quiet labour to protect other mothers from being distracted or frightened.

If you are birthing in a hospital, you automatically become part of that system. A woman's intolerance of labour pain may not be to the pain, but to other people's response to it. A doula told me the following story.

She was with her client in early labour at a particularly conservative hospital. They were strolling down the corridors, looking through the nursery windows at the rows of neatly bundled babies. A nursery nurse popped out the door and upon seeing a woman in early labour blurted out, "When are you gonna get that epidural?" The mother, stunned by this unexpected remark, replied she planned to birth without it.

The nurse retorted, "Oh no you can't do that. Why would you want to? It hurts too much, just have an epidural and enjoy the ride."

Before long, the labouring mother and doula were back in the labour room. Her doctor stopped by to check on her.

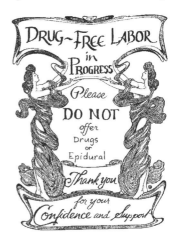

If you like, you could put this kind of sign on your door.

Without discussing the mother's intentions or acknowledging how well she was coping with labour, he asked, "Ready for your epidural? You can have it any time." The mother said she was doing fine, and would like to continue without drugs or anaesthesia. The doctor shook his head as he said, "I don't understand you women who want to birth naturally when there's a better way to do it." Then he disappeared.

During the next eight hours of labour, not one word or gesture of encouragement was offered by hospital staff. All in all, drugs were offered four more times. Were it not for the doula who said "Go for it! You're doing fine," this mother may not have had the personal satisfaction resulting from birthing with strength and self-confidence.

HOW WOMEN COPE WITH PAIN AT HOME

The pain of labour is the same at home as in the hospital. Yet, to get through the pain, women at home rely on different resources than are typically used at the hospital. *How* they do it can be instructive to all expectant mothers, regardless of where they intend to birth.

Women who plan home births are a self-selected group with a clear commitment to labouring drug-free. Knowing that they cannot waiver from that commitment *and* give birth at home, they must envision themselves coping with pain in other ways. They know there will be no "drug net" to fall into when they begin their tightrope walk through labour.

To begin with, a mother's activity is not restricted at home. Being upright and active *significantly* decreases the intensity of pain and may shorten the length of labour. Even though some nurses may encourage walking in the hospital, women often are inhibited or feel restricted by being strapped to a monitor, tied to an IV pole, or limited to pacing in a small room or public hall.

In addition, a woman labouring at home has the freedom to take a warm bath or shower. As the mother relaxes, the effectiveness of contractions increases. More effective contractions mean a quicker labour and an earlier end to pain. (If you are planning to birth in the hospital, ask if baths or showers are available.)

Being confined to a small room can make it seem like pain is filling your whole world. So another advantage a home-birth mother has in dealing with pain is easy accessibility to the outdoors and nature:

trees, clouds, stars or a flower garden are natural distractions during contractions. Feeling cool raindrops or snowflakes, or hearing the singing of birds or the whisper of the wind, are gentle reminders of her connection with nature.

Also significant, though more subtle, is the ongoing infusion of confidence (throughout pregnancy and labour) from a homebirth midwife who routinely attends births where *no* pain medication is used. Women who have chosen home birth not only have a personal relationship with their midwife (whose support they've had throughout pregnancy), but can count on her undivided attention during labour. (There are no disruptive change of shifts at home.) Not even the most compassionate hospital midwives or doctors, simultaneously caring for three, four or five labouring clients (while oppressed by an overwhelming amount of paperwork!) can provide this kind of support.

> "Traditionally, above the head of a Zulu woman of South Africa, is a hole in the roof of her hut where, at night, the stars shine through. She tries to focus on this sky; this is why Zulu women say that in labour they are 'counting the stars with pain.'"[5]

Birthing in privacy, on their own turf, reduces mothers' inhibitions and increases their sense of autonomy. They then feel less self-conscious about doing whatever they need to do. For example, hospitals often discourage, directly or indirectly, groaning, moaning, growling or making other birth sounds. Most home-birth midwives, however, know that primal vocalization helps coping with pain, and encourage women to do *more* of it. The resulting sense of freedom and spontaneity actually facilitates the normal physiological unfolding of labour.

It's not that mothers at home have a higher pain threshold or nerves of steel; they too have fantasies of escaping the pain. But with the unavailability of drugs at home, each contraction forces them to reach deep inside for whatever it will take to meet the challenge. And, most important, their determination is never undermined by well-intentioned offers of relief through drugs or epidurals.

Of course, to continue labouring at home, a mother's labour must be progressing normally. Unusually long and/or abnormal labours are more painful, and erode a woman's ability to cope. In such cases, the wisest and most compassionate care often includes transfer to a hospital for medication to relieve pain, and thereby increase the likelihood of a normal (or less traumatic) birth.

*

WHAT CAN MY PARTNER, BIRTH ATTENDANTS AND I DO TO CREATE A NURTURING ENVIRONMENT?

Two things you can do:

1. SCOUT OUT THE BIRTH TERRAIN

As part of your preparation for birth, research the beliefs and attitudes of your hospital's labour and delivery staff (talk to *several* nurses, midwives, and doctors). Find out how closely their philosophy matches yours *before* you are in labour. You may initially get vague reassurance—"Oh sure, whatever you want is fine." However, the following more specific questions may help you get a truer picture of the system you are about to enter:

- How do nurses (midwives/doctors) at this hospital tend to respond to a woman in pain? What if she is noisy?
- What have you found most useful in helping a woman who doesn't want to use drugs cope with normal pain?
- What do most mothers do to cope with pain (at your hospital)?
- Do you have an anaesthesiologist in the hospital 24 hours a day? How long does it take to get an epidural if I want one? What percentage of mums who deliver here get an epidural? What are the benefits and risks of an epidural?
- Does your hospital or community offer a doula service? Can I bring one with me?

2. HIRE A DOULA

The next chapter explains why hiring a doula is one of the most significant of your pre-birth decisions.

Chapter 37

Don't Give Birth Without A Doula!

I needed my husband there for moral support, but when it came right down to it, I needed to see the doula's face and hear her voice. She was the only one I responded to. We shared a bond She had been right there on that bed before me and had come through it too. I trusted her, and she never let me down.

A MOTHER AND LA LECHE LEAGUE LEADER
QUOTED IN *SPECIAL WOMEN*
BY POLLY PEREZ

In recent years, the tradition of having a doula in birth has been revived. Doula (pronounced doo'-la) is a Greek word meaning "woman who serves." Doulas are trained labour assistants who nurture and assist the labouring and postpartum couple.

Along with nurturance and support, modern doulas offer another important service. When procedures or drugs are being considered, the doula helps parents become an active part of the decision-making process by teaching them to ask the "right" questions. Without adding her own agenda, the skilled doula assists parents in making informed decisions.

Women in labour tend to trust other women, especially those who have given birth. When a father offers his labouring wife empathy, it often feels hollow for her. But when a woman who has experience of labour offers reassurance, it's accepted.

A well-intentioned, compassionate father, who has never seen intense labour pain, might encourage his wife to accept (or request) pain medications or an epidural that she could do without. At the time, the mother may be grateful. Later, however, countless mothers have shared with me their regret, disappointment, or resentment that they didn't get the encouragement they needed to get through that tough point in labour.

Asking your husband to be your sole guide through labour is like asking him to lead the way on a climb of Mt. Everest. He may be smart and trustworthy, you may love him, but in the Himalayas you'd both be a lot better off with a Sherpa!

EVEN IMAGINARY DOULAS CAN HELP

Marci was in the heat of labour when fleeting doubts in her ability to cope with pain began to surface. Nearing the end of labour, Marci was in Labourland's dream-like state when an image of a strong, dark-skinned warrior in a loin cloth, standing on the mesa, her long hair blowing in the wind, first appeared between contractions.

"She 'spoke' to me between contractions, and at the peak of contractions, said, 'Go on, you can go further, you are strong, you can give birth.' And we went further through the hardest part of labour together."

DOULAS HELP FATHERS TOO

I just want it to be my husband and me …
he's been really involved.

VICKY, PREGNANT MUM

*

Why do we need a stranger at our birth?
I'm afraid I'll be left out.

ANTHONY, EXPECTANT FATHER

Imagine being in labour for twelve, sixteen, even twenty-four hours making painfully slow progress. Long labours are exhausting … for everyone. They also create anxiety and raise doubts.

QUESTION: If you brought along your husband or a girlfriend who had never been at a birth, but had taken birthing classes, how do you think he or she would respond to you saying, "I can't do this, do something!"

ANSWER: They'd probably gulp, look worried, and frantically try to think of something helpful to say or do.

Thanks to doulas, we don't have to put our partners in situations like this. Remember, throughout history, it's been experienced mothers who have helped other mothers through labour.

*

WHAT HAPPENS WHEN DOULAS ASSIST THE MOTHER AND FATHER?

NOTE TO READER: *Even if you have an aversion to statistics and have developed an "I'll skip the research" reflex, you'll find it worthwhile to hang in there for the next few pages. I think you'll be amazed by how significant an impact doulas can have on birth and the family.*

A SUMMARY OF THE GROUNDBREAKING HOUSTON STUDY

To investigate the impact of doulas, a large study was conducted at Jefferson Davis Hospital in Houston, Texas (Kennell, et al, 1991).[1] All the mothers in the Houston study were healthy, first-time mothers giving birth at term. There were 412 women randomly assigned to one of two groups.

The first group (212 mothers) were assigned an *active* doula, whose support included touching, suggestions and verbal encouragement. The 200 mothers in the second group were assigned an *observing* doula, who sat quietly in a corner taking notes throughout labour, but did not touch or talk to the mother. The control group consisted of 204 women who birthed at the hospital without a doula. Their birth interventions and outcomes were compared to those of the two doula-assisted groups. Table 37.1 summarizes the results:

TABLE 37.1

	CONTROL (No Doula)	DOULA (Observing only)	DOULA (Active Supporting)
Length of labour *(hrs)*	9.4	8.4	7.4
Epidural	55%	23%	8%
Syntocin—*to augment* labour	43%	32%	17%
Caesarean birth	18%	13%	8%
Forceps	26%	21%	8%

DOULAS STRENGTHEN FAMILY RELATIONSHIPS

In a study of 189 first-time mothers (Hofmeyer, et al, 1991; Wolman, 1993) in Johannesburg, South Africa, researchers investigated how the presence of a doula influences a couple's relationship during and after a birth.

The women, randomly assigned to doula and no-doula groups, reported no significant differences in satisfaction with their partner before or during pregnancy. Immediately after giving birth, however, only 30 percent of women in the no-doula group reported their relationship with their partner was better, while 71 percent of those who were attended by a doula felt their relationship had improved. By six weeks postpartum, 85 percent of the mothers in the doula group reported increased satisfaction with their partners, compared to only 49 percent of the no-doula group.[2,3]

Mothering the mother and father in labour and early postpartum apparently creates a desirable postpartum "halo effect." With the support of a skilled doula, couples experience emotional success in birth, and feel mothered while learning to nurse and care for their new baby. This kind of beginning gives new mothers and fathers a foundation of confidence and good will to build on.

COMMENTS:

1. In the no-doula group only 12 percent delivered naturally (that is, without anaesthesia, medications, or forceps), a striking contrast to the 55% of doula-assisted mothers who had natural deliveries.

2. Even in those labours where doulas were assigned as "observers," meaning they did not touch the mother but stayed in a corner taking notes, labour outcomes improved!

The future well-being of your baby isn't solely determined by medical events surrounding its birth. Its life will be affected dramatically by the quality of its parents' relationship, as well as their perceptions of him or her. Doula-attended births enhance mother-infant bonding, as described in the findings below.

Wolman found that when compared to the no-doula group, mothers who were "mothered" by a doula through labour "were more positive on all dimensions involving specialness, ease, attractiveness and cleverness of their babies." They believed they were closer to their babies and felt they were adapting to motherhood better than did the control group. Doula-attended mothers felt they could take care of their babies better than anyone else, but no-doula mothers believed others could care for their babies as well as they could.[4]

DOCTORS, NURSE-MIDWIVES, NURSES ... AND DOULAS

I couldn't and wouldn't practice obstetrics today without doulas. They give me the confidence of knowing the labouring mother is not frightened or alone, and is always in the capable hands of a professional labour assistant. The quality and continuity of care should not be regarded as a "fringe benefit," "an extra," but as an essential and irreplaceable part of the birthing experience.

HARLAN ELLIS, M.D.
QUOTED IN *SPECIAL WOMEN*
BY POLLY PEREZ

New faces and frequent interruptions can disrupt concentration in labour. During a hospital birth you can expect that at least six unfamiliar people will come in and out of your labour room performing various functions (lab techs, nurses, doctors, students, as well as people from housekeeping and admitting). However, despite these intrusions, the presence of your doula is the continuous thread that you can hold on to throughout your labour.

"I once helped a first-time mother through labour. Near the end of labour, the mum curled up into a squat against a couch. It was apparent she had reached complete dilation and was beginning to push. She told me she could not move to the bed; I called the nurse, who called in the doctor.

The young doctor walked in and gasped when he took in the scene. He looked over at the nurse and said pleasantly, 'We need to get her in the bed. We can't have her pushing on the floor!' I explained to the doctor that the mother had just told me she couldn't get up and move to the bed and that she wanted to deliver her baby right where she was.

The doctor looked at me with a worried expression and said, 'Well, I haven't ever delivered a baby like *this*—in a squat on the floor.' I answered softly, 'That's okay because she never has either.'

We both smiled. He said 'Okay.' And he got down on his knees and attended the birth. It was a beautiful birth."

– CAMERON BENJAMIN,
CERTIFIED DOULA

Unlike nurses or midwives, doulas are not employees of the hospital, and therefore have no other commitments during a woman's labour. This allows a doula to provide one-on-one, continuous labour support (without shift-changes) throughout labour and early postpartum.

Many nurses and midwives wish they could provide more personal bedside support, but the demands on their time make this very difficult. However, once medical personnel see the positive impact doulas have on labouring couples, they become enthusiastic about having another resource which can help couples through labour.

POSTPARTUM: YOU DON'T HAVE TO DO IT ALONE

For many new mothers and fathers, particularly in our mobile society where extended family may be thousands of miles away, the return home following the excitement of birth is often a lonely, overwhelming, and exhausting time. This is another crucial time when mothers (and fathers) need to be mothered; the nurturance they receive helps them nurture their new baby.

Along with the joy and excitement of caring for your new baby, the months following your baby's birth include an emotional minefield: isolation; financial worries; anxiety about baby-care and breastfeeding; changes in your relationship, work and social life; sleep deprivation; loss of spontaneity and freedom.

There's just never enough energy or time to …

* take a nap,
* take a bath,
* tidy up the house,
* make dinner,
* read a book,
* or exercise.

ENTER: THE HOMEVISTING POSTPARTUM DOULA!

The doula can provide invaluable postpartum assistance. She is first and foremost a companion, bringing encouragement, advice and the benefit of experience. Here's a sampling of what doulas can offer:

* Reviewing and working through birth experiences
* Preparing a special herbal bath for the mother, and giving her time to enjoy it
* Massaging her shoulders, feet, or total body
* Preparing a nutritious lunch, or making dinner
* Tidying up the house
* Identifying signs of postpartum depression, early
* Rocking the baby while the mother takes a nap
* Breastfeeding support and consultation
* Teaching cord care and checking for jaundice
* Reassurance and advice about caring for a newborn
* Helping the new family make postpartum connections in the community

MOTHERING THE MOTHER (AND FATHER) STARTS HEALTHIER AND HAPPIER FAMILIES.

HOW TO FIND A PROFESSIONAL DOULA

If you have a midwife she may double as your doula, providing she can be with you without other demands on her time and attention (i.e., you are her *only* client in-labour). However, if your hospital nurse-midwife can't promise continuous, one-on-one care throughout labour, hire a doula.

If you want information about doulas in your area, ask your health care providers, hospital, or contact Doula UK, PO Box 26678, London, N14 4WB (tel: 0871 433 3103; www.doula.org.uk).

If there are no professional doulas where you live, ask an especially caring and nurturing woman, preferably a mother, to assist you. You might suggest she read *Mothering the Mother* by Klaus, Kennel and Klaus, to help her understand her role.[5]

FURTHER INFORMATION

The following websites offer good sources of information on pregnancy and birth in the UK:

Logo for the Art of Birthing Doulas, designed by Ila Nuñez. The heart consists of two women (mother and doula), heads bowed and touching — through the hard work of labour — to produce the flower: the birth of the mother and baby.

www.birthchoice.co.uk
www.homebirth.org.uk
www.independentmidwives.org.uk
www.doula.org.uk
www.aims.org.uk

Chapter 38

Proven Pain Techniques

This chapter presents twelve pain-coping techniques which have been effective for women dealing with the pain of childbirth. The more options you have, the more likely something will work for you. Don't select just a few techniques in advance— the ones you overlook might be the ones that would be most helpful in labour.

IMPORTANT: *Practise techniques frequently to gain mastery.*

Don't be lulled into false confidence if you experience instant success with the techniques. It's not difficult to experience positive results quickly while holding ice sitting in a comfortable chair, in a pain-free body, in a relatively stress-free room! If you stop there and don't practise these techniques in your daily life, you will not master them, and you may be disappointed in them in labour.

When these techniques become a "habit," instead of a "technique," they work better in stressful situations like labour. A thinking or fretful mind will not be helpful in labour, and will interfere with your ability to trust, relax and even breathe calmly. So, it is worthwhile to acquire a new habit of being able to bring yourself back to a quiet, but aware, mind in a stressful situation.

PARTNERS-IN-PAIN

Fathers and birth partners who learn these techniques, holding ice, will not only understand how they work, but also will know what kind of guidance is most helpful while using them.

*

Worksheets to help you learn these pain techniques can be found in Appendix C.

Habits are formed by repetition. Our stressful daily lives, fortunately (or unfortunately), offer hundreds of opportunities to practise (and master) concentration techniques. Being-in-labour is a continuation of your life, not a separate event. Labour is a continuous series of activities, including waves of emotional and physical stress (not just sitting relaxed in a chair). When practise and awareness of breath become part of your moment-to-moment living, it will just continue into the first contraction, and the next … into pushing … into mothering. I suggest two ways to do this:

1. Choose one activity you do every day, such as driving, washing dishes, or preparing food. Make a commitment to practise a technique, wholeheartedly, during that activity for at least five minutes every day. Notice what happens with your breath, emotions, and sensations. Experiment and fine tune the technique until it becomes part of you. If you have a teacher or friends who are experienced in these pain techniques, ask questions if you are having difficulty (so you can master them before labour).
2. Throughout your day, use ordinary emotional and physical pain and stresses to practise a technique that brings you into the moment, into quiet mind and breathing. It's not hard to practise relaxation techniques while you are relatively relaxed sitting in a quiet room. The real challenge, however, is to practise during physical pain (e.g., a headache, backache or yoga class) or emotional pain (e.g., after an argument with your partner or the aggravation of sitting for an hour in a waiting room).

LEARNING WITH ICE CUBES

If you were to practise each of the following techniques without a contrasting sensation of pain, you would find them deeply relaxing; they might even put you to sleep. Although *nothing* can simulate labour pain, I use ice cubes, dubbed "pain cubes," to help people in childbirth classes investigate their responses to pain.

To test the effectiveness of these pain-coping techniques (or your mastery of them), induce an unpleasant sensation (pain) by holding an ice cube in your hand for a 60-second "contraction." If you want a stronger sensation to work with, hold the ice against your wrist or behind your ear.

GETTING YOUR BASELINE RESPONSE TO PAIN

Start by holding an ice cube in your hand while your partner times a 60-second "contraction" for you. Concentrate on feeling the cold, burning, aching sensation of the ice and see how long a minute feels. This experiment works best if you allow yourself to make a fuss about it; complain and whine as much as you need to. Try not to distract yourself, even if you know how.

When your partner announces "time's up," put the ice in a cup and talk about what you noticed. In particular, pay attention to how your mind looked for a way out.

After students in my class have practised the basics of any technique using one ice cube, I challenge them further. Fathers are instructed to hold two ice cubes, one against each of the mother's wrists or behind her ears. This dual locus of pain makes it more difficult to isolate, ignore or escape; to cope, you must immerse your whole body-mind-breath into the technique you are practising.

This also allows fathers insight into their reactions when seeing their partner in pain. With two ice cubes, mothers often lose their composure and rock, breathe harder or complain. Some fathers rise to the occasion with strong, firm encouragement, helping their partners stay focused on the technique, while others become tongue-tied or take the ice off.

1: BREATH AWARENESS

In what way does awareness of breath influence your response to pain?

There is a popular saying, "one day at a time." A "day" is too long when you're in labour, so, experienced midwives often encourage a labouring woman to "take it one contraction at a time."

Most contractions in labour are about a minute long. When you're in pain, a minute can seem a very long time. That's why it may be even more useful to "take it one *breath* at a time."

YOUR BREATHING IS *ALREADY* PERFECT

Be aware of how your breath changes with pain; make no effort to change the natural pattern of your breath. Consider that with all other activities, you trust your body's internal wisdom to adjust your breathing pattern, heart rate, digestive processes, and so on. As pregnancy and labour progress, your body will naturally make necessary physiological adjustments. No conscious thought or effort is necessary. It's already perfect—just notice your perfect breathing pattern.

TRY BREATH AWARENESS:

To find out how this works, take an ice cube in your hand and hold it for a minute. Bring your *full awareness* to your breathing; notice exactly when exhalation begins ... and ends. With utter curiosity, notice how the sensation of the ice changes *as you breathe in and as you breathe out.*

"Is *this* outward breath long or shallow? Is it soft or tight? What is the sound of this breath? What is the feeling in my belly when I breathe out? When does this breath end (or begin)?" (In labour women usually blow the exhalation out slowly, and some-what forcefully, as if blowing a candle flame out).

If you notice your mind begin to wander, get stuck on the sen-sation of ice, or look for a way out ... with the next breath in bring your full attention back to breath awareness. As one mother who mastered this said, "It took a lot of concentration, but if I concentrated intensely on my breathing, I couldn't feel the ice!"

Contrast the difference between holding ice this time and the "getting a baseline" exercise in which you focused on the pain. What happened this time?

Like breath, pain is never static or motionless; it is changing in intensity and location moment-to-moment. Pain comes and goes, but your memory or ideas about pain can become fixed in the mind. A memory doesn't need to be part of your present situation, but when it is, it may dictate what you experience.

Ideas about what pain *should* be, or how you should feel or respond, can overwhelm you. If that happens you will begin looking for a way out, thinking you cannot handle it or fearing it will never end.

The more ideas you bring, the more you will "suffer" and struggle in labour. Try to let go of ideas and just notice what is happening. Don't even substitute "positive" ideas for "negative" ones. Instead, while focusing on your outward breath, substitute pure awareness of breathing for thoughts or judgements about what is unfolding.

*

Breath Awareness is a simple, but powerful exercise. It's so simple that after a few minutes, some people think "Okay I've got this. I've been breathing for years, nothing special about breathing. What's next? Show me something else, something more interesting than watching my breath."

Don't kid yourself. It's not *that* simple!

*

TRY ADDING IMAGINATION TO BREATH AWARENESS:

Your brain will be so busy watching breath and an image, it will have little left to watch the pain. For example, as you breath out ...

- See a flower opening slowly.
- Or with a strong breath out ... imagine your pelvic bones floating apart ... making more room for your baby's head to float downward through the pelvis.
- Watch waves rise and fall as you breathe in ... and out.

Time's up. How did adding imagery change the intensity of the sensation?

2: NON-FOCUSED AWARENESS

Ancient Japanese swordsmen practiced nonfocused awareness of the total moment. They were motivated by knowing that any lapse in concentration could mean a sudden death. Out of the corners of their eyes, samurai warriors might have seen the crowd gathered to watch, but they couldn't *look* at the crowd. Their ears may have heard the crowd, the sounds of birds or of battle all around them, but they could not *listen* to any sound other than those critical to their own survival.

Samurai concentration was fierce; they were totally present, aware of everything but not distracted by anything. If during a duel, a swordsman focused exclusively on his opponent's eyes, he might stumble on uneven ground and lose his footing (as well as his head).

LEARNING FROM THE SAMURAI

One of the best ways of coping with fear, exhaustion and pain in labour is to focus on the immediate situation in its wholeness, rather than letting any isolated, fragment grab your attention. If in labour you focus intensely on just one thing, you will surely miss something else of importance. For example, if you are watching the foetal monitor tracing, you may miss the love in your partner's eyes; if you are dominated by your dread of pain, you may ignore what your body is telling you about its need to change positions (which might actually reduce the pain).

Staying open to *all* sensations, moment-to-moment, removes pain from its central place in your awareness.

> Nearing the end of labour
> I NOTICED long outward breaths
> become a wailing
> that merged with sharp cervical pain.
> At the same time,
> I LISTENED for Little Bird, our parakeet,

TRY NFA:

Find out how Non-Focused Awareness affects your response to pain while holding a piece of ice in your hand for a one-minute "contraction." This can be practised as a solo exercise, or with the help of a partner who can time the "contraction" and guide you.

Non-Focused Awareness means you are open to all of your senses. So, first try keeping your eyes opened slightly, not "looking" around the room for, or at, any thing in particular. Just notice what you are seeing in front of you.

Then, try it again with your eyes closed. What do you see when your eyes are closed? Soft darkness, dream-like imagery?

Which way works best for you?

who had been accompanying my birth song
through each contraction; and
I saw the afternoon winter light
filtering through the blinds;
I smelled the aroma of chocolate birth-day cake baking.
I felt the firm, reassuring touch of my husband's hand on my lower back.

In this multi-layered awareness
I was less self-centred and self-conscious;
and everything around me became part of my
birth.

Next, as you take up the ice …

Bring your full attention to your outward breath.
Then, notice:
What you are seeing …
What you are hearing …
What is touching you and what you are touching …
Notice your emotions …

What you are smelling (the fragrance of herbs, aromatherapy) …

Notice how the sensation is changing with each breath out.

During labour, this step would be included *after* the contraction has peaked.

Continue, in sequence, or randomly, until the minute is up.

*

HERE'S AN EXAMPLE OF NFA:

"I see the sheet … white … wrinkles … shadow.

"I hear my breathing … clock ticking … crickets … bus.

"Hand on leg … my belly rising as I breathe in … melting ice trickling through my fingers.

"I see white … wrinkles … shadows … hear voices … crickets … breathing … knees on the floor … white … shadows … white …"

FURTHER INSTRUCTIONS

DON'T THINK, DON'T JUDGE

NFA works best when you simply experience what you are aware of—without any conscious reflection or judgement about it. The moment you begin thinking, evaluating, labelling (good/bad; I want more/less/none) you forfeit the benefits of this exercise, and your pain will return to its original intensity.

EMBRACE DISTRACTIONS

In every labour there are bound to be "distractions" (e.g., ringing telephones, machines beeping or people talking).

Unplug the phone, close the hall door and make every effort to eliminate unwanted disturbance. Even so, the machines may beep, an IV may need to be started or a car alarm may scream into your consciousness.

You can't control your environment, but you can use the practice of NFA to assimilate these distractions constructively and thereby change their *meaning*.

AVOID "FEELING"

Mothers have taught me that when cued to "notice what you are feeling," they get stuck in the pain of the ice (or contractions). That cue also guides them into their emotions rather than sensations (which are the focus of this practice). Therefore, it's best to avoid focusing on what you are "feeling." Instead, be aware of the sensations of breathing, seeing, hearing, smelling and what's touching you (e.g., a breeze, someone's hand on your back or floor under your feet).

*

NFA Variations

A: VERBAL/NON-VERBAL SHIFTING

- Say silently to yourself what you are noticing
- Say aloud what you are noticing
- Listen to cues from your birth partner as you:
  Notice silently or
  Say aloud what you're noticing

B: QUAKER LISTENING

A few years ago, a parent in childbirth class taught this meditative-concentration technique, and it's become a favourite. Taking up the ice cube, listen to your partner's hypnotic cadence suggesting the following:

Bring your full attention to your next outward breath.
Notice what you are hearing just outside your ears …
The sounds at the edge of the room … in the next room …
just outside the building, on the street …

With your next breath, notice the sounds on the street …
just outside the window … in the other room …
in this room … right next to you …
maybe even listen within …
Let go of the ice (pain) with the next outward breath.

AN EXAMPLE OF QUAKER LISTENING

I hear my breathing …
My partner's breathing …
Voice … silence … fan …
Rain on the window …
Thunder …
Car …
Rain drops …
Footsteps …
Sheets rustling …
Breathing …
Silence.

CUEING INSTRUCTIONS FOR NFA

1. Speak slowly, allowing her to listen for a full breath or two, before offering a new suggestion.
2. If there is a distracting noise when you are suggesting she notice the sounds in the room, include the distracting noise, too, like this: "Notice the sounds in this room and on the street …"
3. Give *general* suggestions rather than specific. "Notice the sounds coming from the hall" rather than "Notice the beeper …"

ADDITIONAL OBSERVATIONS:

Don't expect to use one technique continuously throughout labour. The mind can't concentrate that intensely for hours on end. Try different techniques, or turn to Non-Focused Awareness to help centre your attention. Sometimes just coast in Breath Awareness.

INTERNAL MONOLOGUE

WITHOUT NFA	WITH NFA
Oh no, another one (contraction)	*I notice tightening (uterine)*
I don't want to do this anymore	... hear outward breath
It's taking too long	... hear voices, breath ...
Don't talk ...	... voices ... silence
Stop that beeping	... beep ... silence ... beep
Close that door ...	(feel, hear) Long breath out
I can't concentrate ...	See door opening
Shut that machine up	Hear beep ... paper crinkling

With practise, Non-Focused Awareness becomes non-verbal. You will observe or experience without labelling, flowing from one modality to another, always aware of your breath.

Mums have told me it's more difficult to practise NFA in a very quiet room, or in a hospital room with unfamiliar or disturbing sounds. They find it easier when listening to tapes of music or nature sounds.

Without any conscious effort, breathing becomes slow and rhythmical when the mind is focused. Steady breathing in turn calms the mind and allows for better concentration. Sometimes mothers in labour hyperventilate (fast, shallow breathing) which causes dizziness and numbness in the hands. It is not possible to hyperventilate or hold your breath while using this technique. Try it and see.

*

TROUBLESHOOTING

If while practising NFA or any variation, you rated the sensation above a five on your worksheet, these questions and tips might help:

Q: Are you looking around too actively for new things to see?
A: "Looking" often weakens concentration and intensifies pain. Keep your eyes at rest, focused on what's in your natural line of vision.

Q: Are you analyzing or judging?
A: Intensify your concentration, leaving no room for other thoughts or judgements.

Q: Are you losing your train of thought or are you easily distracted?
A: Have someone cue you through the "contraction."

Q: Is your stream of awareness flowing too rapidly or too slowly?
A: Change your pace. Often during intense pain, going faster eliminates the space to think or worry. Or focus on one sensation (e.g., Quaker Listening).

*

SIMPLY OBSERVING, WITHOUT JUDGING, BRINGS SUCCESS

When Brooke first tried Non-Focused Awareness she complained that the technique didn't work for her. So we investigated what had happened. During the exercise a low flying airliner passed over the office. Here's what she was saying to herself:

"I hear the loud airplane. Why do they have to fly so low? When are they gonna finish that new runway? That sound drives me crazy.

That's *not* Non-Focused Awareness! Brooke lost track of what this exercise required and she reverted to a more typical inner chatter about her *reactions* to what was going on.

After reviewing the importance of simply observing without judgement, Brooke tried it again. Fortunately, another plane flew over the office, and this time Brooke succeeded at keeping her sensory channels open and her thought channel closed:

"I hear a plane approaching. I hear birds singing … a dog bark. I hear the airplane … louder, I hear the engine-sound fading."

This time, Brooke reported she was completely unaware of any discomfort in her hand holding the ice. What was different? The difference was no judging, no reacting and hearing all sounds with equal awareness.

HOW FATHERS USE NON-FOCUSED AWARENESS IN LABOUR

Attending labour is initially exciting, but often becomes tedious and exhausting. It's not unusual to want to check-out or to start worrying.

Fathers practising NFA during labour will be more aware of their partners' needs, and feel more present and calm at the birth of their child.

NON-FOCUSED AWARENESS FOR LIFE

You can practise non-focused awareness just about anywhere, anytime—in your stuffed chair, while washing the dishes or while falling asleep. Non-focused awareness clears the mental fog that shrouds your own experience of day-to-day living.

Mothers praise how this exercise helps them overcome minor aches, discomforts, and insomnia during pregnancy. Practising non-focused awareness during sleep-deprived and frazzled postpartum days is soothing, and heightens your connection with your baby during ordinary moments like changing a dirty nappy.

*

3: EDGES:

"Into the destructive element, immerse yourself."

JOSEPH CONRAD

The more actively we try to push away a sensation or feeling, the more dominating it becomes. The Edges technique advocates "making friends" with pain. By getting to know pain better, the added tension and fear created by resisting it recede. Less tension and fear means less pain.

Rather than trying to push away or "distract" yourself from pain, be utterly curious about it. Pain is not static, but our memory of it is. Once we memorize the sensation, its location, and even the meaning we give it, we are responding to its "history," rather than what it *is* in the moment. Even when it changes (and it does moment-to-moment), we don't notice the difference. Our responses get stuck on what used to work (or didn't), instead of what could be working best now.

The experience of ongoing, intense pain exhausts and overwhelms our mind and, in time, makes pain seem unmanageable. During those periods pain can define our whole being. Opening our mind to each sensation, and discovering where it begins and ends, actually reduces its psychological size and makes it less frightening. This perceptual leap is a significant first step in managing pain, but requires courage.

VARIATIONS OF EDGES

A: EDGES OF COMFORT

Some people see their cup half full, others half empty. Another kind of edge to notice in labour is the edge of *comfort*.

Hold an ice cube in your hand or against your wrist (Change hands when practising more than one variation).

TRY EDGES:

Hold an ice cube in your hand, or against your wrist for a 60-second "contraction."

*Immerse yourself
into an exploration
of the sensation.
As you breathe out ...
Be curious: What is
this moment's pain?
Notice exactly where
it begins and ends ...
How its location
and intensity
change.
As you breathe out ...*

Repeat the exploratory sequence until the "contraction" is over.

Bring your full awareness to your first outward breath …
Ask yourself "Where exactly is the edge of comfort? …
Notice where your body is soft and relaxed …
And comfortable (pain free).
With each breath out …
Bring your full attention to where your body isn't hurting …

B: SEEING THE EDGE OF PAIN UNDER A MAGNIFYING GLASS

Take up another piece of ice.

Imagine looking at the sensation through a magnifying glass, and being really curious while slowly, carefully, studying its parameters, millimetre by millimetre.

With each breath out … notice
details like:
Colours … Textures … Crevices,
cracks or smooth edges …
Is the border solid, rigid or flexible, misty, watery ? …
With each breath out …
Move the magnifying glass again and …
Continue to notice the subtle changes in the
living border of pain.

C: SOFTENING AROUND THE EDGES: A GUIDED VISUALIZATION

Even if you are able to master these exercises quickly now, it's more difficult to maintain necessary concentration in the midst of labour's exhaustion. It may be easier during a painful contraction if someone talks you through it. Practising this variation with your partner will help prepare you to work together in labour:

Mother holds a piece of ice.

*

BIRTH PARTNER CUES: As soon as the "contraction" starts, begin speaking in a slow, rhythmic cadence, in synch with her breath (so she has time to absorb what you are saying and do what you are suggesting):

Bring your full awareness to your next outward breath …
[as she breathes in say]
With your next breath out soften …
all around …
the edges of the sensation …
[as she breathes in say:]
Imagine all the muscles, ligaments …
even the bones near the pain … [as she breathes out]
… soften, melt away …
That's right … let the sensation and everything around it melt and
fade away.

*

The timing of the suggestions is particularly important because a woman
in Labourland needs time to absorb the meaning of your directions. On
the in-breath, *prepare* her for what she will do on the out-breath.

*

Repetition is soothing. Use the same imagery or adjectives throughout a contraction (continue for about six contractions). Women in
labour don't need creative variations, they need to master concentration. Repetition can help them do that.

These suggestions may be helpful:

> soften release melt open let go yield blend fall away make room
> make more space flow with it

4: FINDING THE CENTRE OF PAIN

See what happens when you bring your attention from the edges
directly into the *centre* of the sensation. In this exercise, notice how
the centre is not fixed. It moves, sometimes subtly, sometimes rhythmically, fast, or slowly—keep your attention on the moving centre.

When I practice the Centre technique, I think of a hurricane. The
eye of a hurricane is still, while the destructive, forceful winds swirl
around it. When you concentrate on the centre of a sensation, you
may be surprised by the absence of pain (until your mind remembers
the pain, looks for it, and finds it!).

TRY CENTERING:

Hold a piece of ice (or two) for a 60-second "contraction" and:

Bring your full attention to your outward breath ...
As you breathe into the sensation ...
Find its centre ...
With each breath out notice how both the centre ...
and the sensation ...
are in constant movement
Focus your mind's eye on the centre ...

Sometimes the sensation's centre and movement is in synch with your breath. If the sensation increases on the in-breath, imagine suspending the movement or shrinking the centre until you begin your exhalation. Experiment until you find what works for you.

*

5: SPIRALLING

Spiralling suggests opening and expanding, which is perfect for labour. (In fact, some women prefer contractions be called "expansions" to remind them that the work of contractions and pain *is opening* their cervix and bones to release the baby.)

WHAT DOES YOUR SPIRAL LOOK LIKE?

Some people have found it helpful to have soft, loose spirals, like drawing a spiral in the sand with a big stick or a glowing neon light. (For many people, thin line spirals don't seem to be as effective.) Notice how the speed, as well as the tightness of the coiling, affects the sensation.

TRY SPIRALLING:

Hold a piece of ice.

Breathe into the centre of the sensation.

As you breathe out ...
Imagine sending (blowing)
a spiral from the centre
(of the sensation) outward ...

The slower you breathe out
(pushing the spiral with your breath)
the further you spiral away
from the sensation.

WHAT HAPPENS TO YOUR SPIRAL WHEN YOU BREATHE IN?

You might wonder "Should my spiral pause? expand? or move inward?" Apparently, what is most helpful varies from person to person. Experiment, and use what works best.

If the direction you are spiralling in isn't working, try changing the direction. That could mean either using a different plane (horizontal or vertical) or spiralling from the outside into the centre.

*

6: BUILDING A PARTNERSHIP WITH YOUR BABY

Years ago, Daphne, a woman in my childbirth class, told me how before falling asleep she would sit in bed, rub her belly and talk to her baby, "Please don't hurt mummy too much, please come out quickly because mummy is afraid of the pain …" Later, she attributed her fast, strong labour and success in handling labour pain to her baby's cooperation; it helped them bond right from the start.

A year later, an expectant mother told me how, after hearing Daphne's story, she began imagining a joint effort with her baby. She fantasized what it might be like to be born, and wanted to make it quick and painless for her baby. She also imagined the baby helping *her* during labour. She murmured to her baby about coming out: "Hurry up and come out. I want to see you, I can't wait to meet you … Let's work hard together so we can finally meet."

I was intrigued by these women's experiences and spent some time reflecting on how their establishing an emotional partnership with their babies might have helped them with the pain and hard work of labour. One way of conceptualizing these stories is that they were pre-labour self-hypnotic inductions. By establishing and practising this playful way of thinking about getting their baby out, the mothers unconsciously laid down positive tracks about a cooperative, loving relationship with their baby during labour.

Mental exhaustion and discouragement are more likely to occur when a person feels isolated during a difficult task. In the midst of your deepest withdrawal into labour, the intense, close physical relationship between you and your baby is different from the contact of a loving husband or caring birth attendant. Having the image of a loving little partner going through labour with you creates the possibility of feeling shared effort, purpose and connection.

Building a partnership with your baby may soothe and comfort you in ways that actually help your body open to birth. In any case, you can have fun practising this!

*

7: FINDING YOUR VOICE

Living in the Southwest has influenced our childbirth classes. Picture this: Mothers sitting in a circle on the floor, learning to labour-howl while a tape of howling coyotes fills the room. Later, fathers join the circle for co-chanting. Some people start out a bit inhibited, but once they warm up, it isn't easy getting them to stop.

A widely accepted (though disastrously misleading) notion is that all women should respond to labour pain in the same way: quietly. Ironically, this usually means behaving in a most unnatural way: breathing in controlled, stylized patterns; refraining from moaning or wailing; and lying still rather than writhing or rocking. Sounds which suggest the sexual nature of birth may subtly be shaped out of a woman's repertoire.

Yet many women have confided that one of the unexpected gifts of labour was finding their "voice." Perhaps it was the first time in their lives they said, "No," "Stop it," "Don't touch me, go away" or simply screamed primitively. (This may be the first, but not the last, time they'll be screaming in motherhood.) At other times, the primal instinct to protect and nurture their newly born forced them to be assertive, ask questions or say no. These women have found their voice.

This does not mean that every woman needs to be vocal in labour. Working with thousands of women has taught me that women who are naturally quiet and introspective are more likely to be quiet (without any special effort) in labour. Women who are verbally expressive every day of their lives are *naturally* that way in labour, too.

Birth customs and attitudes about vocalization have their own idiosyncratic roots (both individual and cultural). Sometimes those expectations, both internal and external, script and suppress a woman's vocalization in labour.

Be aware of scripts: approach your birth with an openness to do whatever your body needs you to do. Don't make a prideful plan to labour quietly; that might not be you.

When you hit your thumb with a hammer, you probably say "Ouch!" or chant some profanity. Guys in my classes who work in construction often playfully ridicule the notion of stoically and quietly breathing through that kind of pain. They know that vocalization through pain can be both a distraction and a release.

In labour, it's as though a *cervix* has something to say about its incredible stretching and opening: perhaps, "ouch, o o u u c h, O o o u u u u u u u h!," or sometimes the sound is a deep, long moaning: "A a a a a a h h h … O o o o o o o o w w. A mother might give the baby moving orders, like: "Baby come out … " or "Baby get out, baby get out B a b y G e t O o o o u u u u u u t! …

Another may talk to her cervix, saying: "Cervix open, open, open,

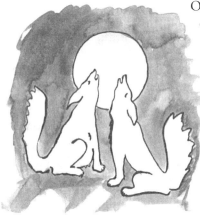

Oooooooooopen, Ooooo ooooopen, open cervix, open, open." Of course, to say this, she simultaneously must be visualizing her cervix opening in her mind. I also suggest that women visualize their cervix softening and opening with each painful contraction, while chanting such things as, "Open like a flower, flower of life. Open like a flower, flower of love."

Other kinds of chants, which are common, though less poetic, may be along the lines of "!*@>…&h#^…%@#df?*t!…" Remember, strong labour requires power and aggression (which increases oxytocin). A string of profanity for some women may reconnect them with their forceful core, and help nature take its course.

All these chants are empowering and effective because they unify body-mind, leaving no room for doubt, fear, or self-pity. Whatever the sounds or words are, their uninhibited, complete expression merges with the pain and momentarily dissipates it. Vocalization in labour is primordial, beautiful, and it works.

As you get closer to pushing, moaning or chanting gradually turn into guttural growling (at the peak of contractions). In labour, women are rarely aware of this. But when midwives or nurses hear it, they realize it is the early sound of pushing. When they ask mothers, "Are you pushing?" or "Was that a push?," they often don't know. The body, in its wisdom, has begun pushing without any conscious intention. Soon after, the mother realizes she *is* pushing!

*

When a mother wants to keep the pain to a level she can manage *without making noise*, the Mind sends Body an urgent message: "Wait! Slow down!" Fear of pain, of losing control, or of being unladylike stimulates the release of adrenalin, which slows down labour. Labour pain may remain "manageable" but the labour process will take a longer time.

As I write this, I recall a story I heard in a childbirth class. After I had described the importance of primal vocalization (and given a live demonstration of it), Zena, one of the mothers, wondered whether this explained what might have happened to her sister's labour a few years earlier:

> My sister was in good, strong labour and labour had been progressing well. Nearing the end of labour, she was about seven centimetres dilated ... she began wailing and moaning through contractions, on her hands and knees, just like you showed us. Her nurse came in and said, "I'm sorry, but you're making the doctor nervous. Try to be quiet."
>
> My sister managed to be quiet, but soon after her labour petered out. The birth changed directions. After labour slowed down, she was given pitocin, which led to an epidural. And we always wondered what happened.

Of course, there are many factors which might cause a labour to slow down. Mothers and midwives have told me that a woman who feels free to follow her natural patterns of breathing and vocalization does better in labour.

WHAT THE BIRTH-COMPANION CAN DO:

• If you are in a hospital, close the door.

If the people working with you are uncomfortable with natural birth sounds and are telling her to be quiet, or that making noise wastes energy:

• Tell them this is helping her,
• Get a different nurse or
• Send your decibel-sensitive friends or relatives to lunch.

When talking about this in class one night, a father suggested that if people are giving a mum a hard time about being too noisy, cheerfully offer them a deal: if they can be quiet while you pull one of their arms out of its socket, you'll try to make the mum be quiet.

   If the mum is crying out in a high-pitched wail, or it sounds like fear caught in the throat, she may be self-conscious or afraid of letting her pain show. Here's what you can do to encourage her: Say softly, "What's that sound? Make it a little louder … and longer so I can really hear the sound of birth … " or "That sound is good … It means the baby is coming soon. Make the sound deeper, let it come from your belly" (sometimes it helps to model deeper, slower, moaning or chanting).

CO-CHANTING

If the mother begins moaning or chanting words in a rhythmical way, learn her sound and begin co-chanting. This can provide incredible validation and eliminate self-consciousness (especially in a hospital).

Let the sound emerge from the mother. Don't tell her what sound to make or what to chant. (After all, the "right" sound is coming from *her* cervix, not yours.)

Only one person at a time in the room should co-chant. When you co-chant, match her sound, intensity, and volume as closely as possible. If you start before or after, or if you're louder or quieter, it could throw off her concentration.

Be Aware: Sometimes fathers and relatives become so uncomfortable and distressed by raucous vocalization that not only may they anxiously communicate a "Shh-shh, calm down" message, but they may also directly, or indirectly, encourage accepting drugs ("We'll all feel better").

8: THE COMMUNICATION OF TOUCH

How does being held or massaged affect your response to pain?

Some people want to be held and stroked during painful experiences, while others handle pain better when left alone. Regardless of your usual inclination, your needs in labour could be exactly opposite.

TRY TOUCH RELAXATION:

MOTHERS

Most women like to have their lower back, inner thighs or the palm of one hand stroked during contractions. Tell your partner which one of these areas you have chosen for this practise session. If possible, try out other areas to see how each feels.

Hold an ice cube in your hand.

Exhale audibly so your partner can be attuned to your breathing pattern and will know when to stroke. In active labour your breathing (exhalation) will be audible without you making any special effort.

Try to be simultaneously aware of your breathing, being stroked, and the changing sensation of ice melting in your hand.

Afterwards, talk about what worked. If the stroke felt too soft or deep, or the timing was off, try it again.

BIRTH PARTNER

You will need to time a 60-second "contraction;" announce when it begins and ends, or silently indicate this by giving, then taking, an ice cube.

Pay close attention to her breathing pattern. As she breathes out, use a downward stroke matching the length of her exhalation. When she breathes in, lift (or almost lift) your hands off her body, moving them back to your starting point. Then stroke downward as she begins her outward breath.

Your stroke should reflect the intensity of her breathing: When she exhales forcefully at the peak of the contraction, stroke down a bit more firmly; as the contraction wanes and breathing becomes quiet, stroke gently. In this way, your touch mirrors both the speed and intensity of her breath.

If her breathing remains fast or frenzied even after the peak of a contraction, you can help her breathe more slowly and easily by *gradually* slowing down your strokes. Or ask her to breathe out into your hand, which is first placed firmly over her heart, then over her diaphragm, and with the third breath, over her lower belly. Women in labour respond very well to this.

Very often when a labouring woman snaps, "Don't touch me!" what she means is "Don't touch me *that* way." Women in labour generally prefer a firm, sure touch. Featherlight, rapid, nervous rubbing back and forth is likely to stimulate the famous laboursmack or "Don't touch me!" response.

9: A CHOCOLATE BIRTHDAY CAKE

An ordeal during a previous labour often leaves a woman vowing she'll never go through *that* again. Unresolved fear and loss of confidence may unnecessarily narrow what she sees as her range of options during her next pregnancy. She neither trusts her body (it didn't work the first time), nor the medical model (did it rescue her from a crisis or create the crisis?).

After a birth trauma, a woman has a tendency to think in extremes. On the one hand, she may pursue excessive prenatal testing, premature pain relief or rush to an early, even scheduled, Caesarean. On the other hand, she frantically may avoid medical intervention no matter how helpful, or even necessary.

*

When I became pregnant for the second time I realized I was terrified of another long labour. Like other women traumatized by birth, I was unable to trust myself or the medical model. Although I hoped for a natural labour at home, I was trying to accept the possibility of giving birth by Caesarean.

A woman who felt pressured or rushed in a previous labour might respond favourably to the suggestion that she "take all the time in the world" to birth her next baby. But for me (having endured a two-day labour previously), setting a time limit and being receptive to intervention, even a Caesarean if necessary, reflected my openness to whatever would unfold.

One of my most important tasks of preparation was to consider all my options. How long is *too* long in labour? How long could I give myself wholeheartedly to labour pain? How much time was needed to give labour a chance?

My answer hovered around six to eight hours. More than eight hours, I would worry I was "stuck" again. As I was already beginning to accept the possibility of needing another Caesarean, I wanted it sooner rather than later this time.

How would I know it was time to get medical help? In wanting to escape the linear confines of clock-time, I moved to a rounder, sweeter dimension by making up this self-hypnotic jingle:

I will only be in labour as long as it takes
To Make, Bake, Cool, and Frost a Chocolate Cake.

My friend, Janey, was delighted when I asked her to make the chocolate birth-day cake (from scratch) for me in labour. When I attended her birth four years earlier, we made chocolate truffles. Since then we probably have consumed a ton of chocolate together.

Janey arrived about an hour after my labour began. She got right to work making that cake, and every so often I remember hearing a progress report on the cake. The aroma of chocolate baking filled the house. My eight-year-old son, Sky, helped to frost the cake as I crawled in slow motion negotiating the eight-foot hallway between the bathroom and Luc's nursery-to-be.

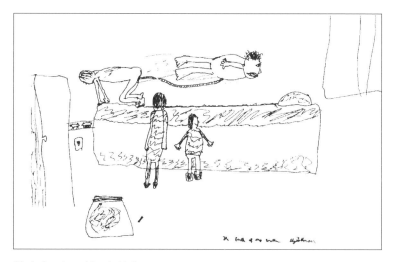

Sky's drawing of Luc's birth

"The pillow is where he's going to land so he doesn't get hurt. The bed is really big and covered with soft covers.

"I am feeling happy—it shows on my face. Luc is freaked out—it's his first time on earth and he's flying, seeing things. Rob is feeling happy and mum is glad."

Soon I heard Janey announce that the cake was done! I looked up and saw her proudly holding up the cake. No sooner had the thought drifted across my mind,"How did she bake the cake so quickly?" than I was swept away by another contraction, and another. Twenty minutes later, Luc was born.

One of the fondest memories of my life is that of Janey, Sky, Rob and me sitting around the pretty Christmas tree, with our midwife, eating the most delicious chocolate birth-day cake I have ever tasted, with newly born Luc bundled in his Butterfly quilt.

HERE'S HOW TO CREATE YOUR OWN SELF-HYPNOTIC JINGLE:

Begin by stating a particular behaviour, belief, or outcome you want to bring about.

Express what you hope for simply and directly. Say what you *do* want, rather than what you don't want. For example, Nikki made up this jingle: "I am a big, strong birthing machine," rather than telling herself, "I'm scared stiff."

Use your sense of humour (and the playful side of being a mother).

Repetition moves the new idea from your left brain to your right brain, and down into your body.

Rhythmical jingles that evoke vivid imagery activate your right brain and thus directly affect your body.

10: MAKING IT STRONGER

When labour seems "stuck" or the mother's confidence and energy are waning, there are several approaches which may help to get things going: changing position, walking, nipple stimulation (which releases oxytocin), warm showers or baths, more fluids (or an IV). If these less interventive efforts don't make a difference, syntocin and epidural may become necessary. Before accepting medical interventions, try this technique. You will need guidance and support from your doula or birth companion and about thirty minutes to get results.

BIRTH COMPANION, DO THIS:

Ask the mother to imagine or pretend she could rate the strength of the contractions from 1 to 10. (Interestingly, in stuck labours, however painful, women do not begin with ten. They often start with 6 or 7.)

Let's say she rated it a "seven." Before the next contraction begins, encourage her to have a real strong "seven" contraction the next time, and to notice what a "seven" (contraction) feels like.

After the contraction is over, ask her if it was a good "seven." If she reports it was, tell her, "On the next contraction, see if you can make it a seven-and-a-half, a real strong 7.5."

After a few of these, say, "I'm wondering what an 'eight' would look like, or feel like. See if you can make this an 'eight.' Strong, steady contractions are bringing your baby home ... Wow! That was a great 'eight.' Do another, maybe an 'eight-and-a-quarter,' but not more than that. Just take it easy, a little bit at a time ... "

When women "control" and become curious about their pain, they concentrate better and relax. This often brings a change in their labour pattern and progress. If this doesn't work, she may truly be "stuck" and then you can try other things to get labour going (e.g., artificially rupturing the membranes, stripping the membranes, an IV, pain-relieving drugs or syntocin).

11. HOT AROMATHERAPY PACKS

A recent (and immediately popular) addition to the pain-coping repertoire offered during Birthing From Within classes is Hot Aromatherapy Packs. This technique was inspired by seeing a photograph of an African mother labouring in front of her birth hut, being

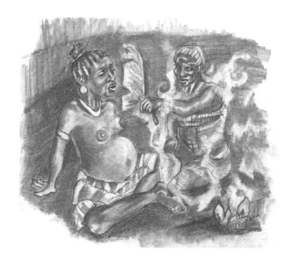

warmed by a glowing fire. Remember, mothers need to be warm in labour; when the room is cold (as it often is in the hospital), mothers are cold. To produce heat, the body releases adrenalin, which as we have already explained, neutralizes oxytocin.

A mother can take a warm bath or shower when available (if she feels up to it). But, when hospitals don't offer this option, or she's not able to get up, hot aromatherapy packs are a perfect solution.

The scent is not only soothing, but adds a pleasant sensation for women to focus on, and most importantly, it gently shifts the mood from the medical to the sensual. As numerous mothers and fathers in my classes have observed, this nurturing labour "ritual" imbues both their inner and outer space with a natural serenity. Fathers seem to enjoy becoming involved in actively nurturing their wives, while mothers soften and open.

HERE'S WHAT YOU'LL NEED:

A 3–5 litre crockpot or a litre-sized electric teapot. Tap water in most hospitals is not very hot to begin with, and will cool quickly in a basin. Even if a nurse offers to microwave a litre of water (which takes 10–15 minutes), when it cools you'll have to call the nurse and wait again. Having to use cool washcloths while waiting for more hot ones defeats the whole idea.

4–6 thick washcloths or cloth nappies. Thick material will hold the heat longer than will thin hospital washcloths.

Aromatherapy Oil: Lavender, Rose Geranium, and/or Ylang Ylang are recommended for labour.

WHAT TO DO

1. If you are birthing in a hospital, you may need to have the electric cord on your crockpot or teapot inspected and approved by the engineering department as a fire-safety precaution. Do this before labour.
2. Heat a litre of water in the crockpot or teapot. The crockpot continually heats the water (if you keep the lid on) while simultaneously serving as your basin. If you decide to use an electric teapot, pour the heated water into a basin, and begin heating another pot of water.
3. Add a capful of aromatherapy oil to the heated water.
4. Soak the washcloths, wring one out at a time and place it on the lower abdomen, and/or thighs or lower back.
5. If you are practising this before labour, mothers should hold an ice cube during "contractions."
6. Remind the mother to focus on Breath Awareness, NFA, and/or your massage. Mothers like it when I suggest they imagine the aromatherapy scent as a safe anaesthetic they can breathe in— and absorb through the skin—in just the right amount, and that *this* anaesthetic can't reach the baby.
7. After every contraction or two, exchange the cool wash cloth for a hot one. Don't disturb the mother's concentration by exchanging washcloths *during* a contraction.
8. Add more aromatherapy oil as needed.

You can buy (or make) microwavable rice or aromatherapy heat packs (they look and feel like bean bags) that provide dry heat for about 30 minutes. There are also commercial (gel) microwavable heat packs that work well.

*

HOT SOCKS

Fill two or three white tube socks with about 2-½ cups of rice or barley, enough to make a supple pack that can hold heat for 20 minutes. Sew or secure the end with a rubberband. Microwave one sock for about two to three minutes.

For an aromatherapy hot pack, add ¼ to ½ cup of dry lavender or chamomile leaves, and/or 4–5 drops of the same essential oils.

12. TRANSCUTANEOUS ELECTRICAL NERVE STIMULATION (TENS)

TENS, with no side effects, is a safer alternative to drugs and helps enhance a mother's feeling of control. It can be used in conjunction with the other pain techniques taught in this chapter (and analgesics if you need them). A TENS unit is a simple device which can be used at home or in the hospital; you can learn to use it during one training session.

There's no consensus in the research literature about the exact mechanism through which TENS alleviates pain. However, some things are known. Pain conduction, like all nerve conduction, is an electrochemical event. When this conduction is interrupted (either by drugs or direct electrical stimulation), the experience of pain is decreased. TENS also has been found to increase endorphin levels in the central nervous system.

In labour, TENS has been found to be particularly helpful to women with back pain, allowing them to stay up and be active. Mums

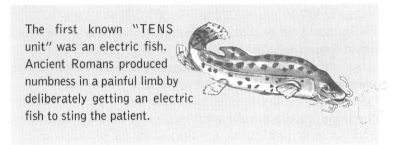

The first known "TENS unit" was an electric fish. Ancient Romans produced numbness in a painful limb by deliberately getting an electric fish to sting the patient.

with an overwhelming fear of being able to cope with pain, especially after a previous negative experience in labour, should consider renting a TENS unit.

HOW EFFECTIVE AND SAFE IS TENS IN LABOUR?

Reviewing nine different studies on obstetric use of TENS, Heywood and Ho (1990) concluded "safety has been confirmed, pain relief has been variable, labours have sometimes been shorter, and most mothers have been very satisfied retrospectively with their labors."[1]

In one study (Harrison, et al, 1986) involving 150 randomly-assigned women, neither midwives nor mothers knew whether a real or placebo TENS unit was being used. Significantly fewer women using real TENS needed analgesia or epidural anaesthesia to complete their labours. In addition, postnatal assessment of pain relief was more favourable among mothers (and their midwives) who had used real TENS machines.[2]

HOW MUCH PETHIDINE IS A TENS UNIT WORTH

One study (Tawfik, et al, 1982) found TENS in labour to be statistically comparable to an average total dose of 93.6 mg of Pethidine. However, TENS mothers did not experience the side effects (nausea, vomiting, or drowsiness), which were reported by 27 percent of the mothers who had used Pethidine.[3]

TENS should not be used during a bath or shower, or if you have a demand-type cardiac pacemaker.

Sometimes TENS units interfere with electronic foetal monitoring when an *internal* foetal scalp electrode is used. It almost never causes interference when an external foetal monitor is used. Interference seems dependent upon particular combinations of monitors and TENS machines, so the problem may never be encountered in some hospitals.[4]

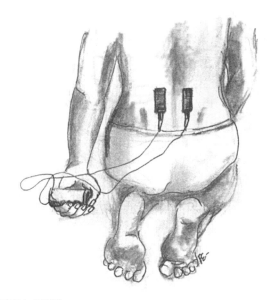

WHAT YOU'LL NEED:

Ask your obstetric physiotherapist or midwife if a TENS unit is available, otherwise you can rent one from the variety of companies specialising in pregnancy and birth care products, or possibly from your childbirth teacher. (I rent TENS units to parents in my Birthing From Within childbirth classes.)

HOW TO USE A TENS UNIT:

Learn to use your TENS unit before labour.

When labour starts, have someone place the electrode pads on your sacral area (You should learn exactly where to place them when you rent your TENS unit). Depending on where you place them, you will affect the nerves serving the uterus, cervix, and/or vagina and perineum.

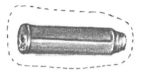

A FINAL WORD: For our readers who are more traditional or stoic in their approach to managing pain, we've included an additional aid. Feel free to cut it out on the dotted lines, and bite as needed.

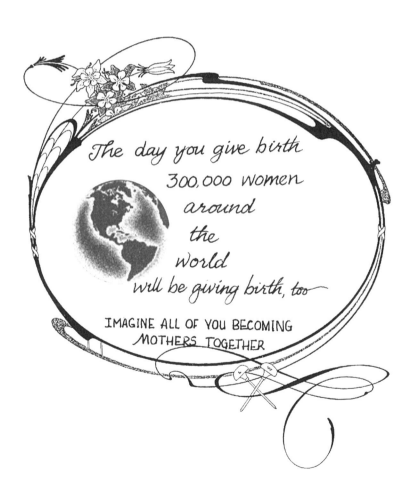

Chapter 39

The Compassionate Use of Drugs and Epidurals

The intention of this chapter is to provide information to
help you make informed choices at your birth, and to reduce
the chance that you'll wind up saying, "If only I had known."

Labour pain is so intense that it's hard for most women to resist
drugs when they're offered. This is especially true near the end of
labour, just before it's time to push. The goal of this chapter is to help
you discriminate between when drugs or an epidural may be genuinely helpful, from the times when they add unnecessary risk and
stress, and wind up being a choice you will regret later.

HOW PAIN HELPS YOU GET YOUR BABY OUT

Nature's blueprint for women giving birth includes pain, and this
pain is purposeful. Pain is experienced when stretch receptors in the
dilating cervix send signals to your brain, calling for more oxytocin to
be released—which in turn fuels labour and increases dilation. The
sensations you're experiencing are part of an ingenious feedback
mechanism which is essential to normal labour and birth.

   The pain and sensations of labour tell you what position is best for
you and how to move in labour to get your baby out. With an
epidural, this feedback is wiped out. Of course, such information
would no longer be useful anyway, because after an epidural you are
immobilized and hooked up to machines (epidural pump, IV and
foetal monitor) and restricted to lying on your back.

   Pain also raises endorphin levels in your body, while analgesic
drugs and epidural anaesthesia lower them. This is significant because
endorphin levels correlate with the release of oxytocin. So, when pain

is relieved through drugs or an epidural, the stimulus for endorphin production is eliminated, and its levels fall. This change is often accompanied by a drop in oxytocin, thus slowing down labour and dilation.

*

Once you're completely dilated, your baby's head will descend deeper and deeper into your pelvis, stretching the muscles in your pelvic floor. This stretching stimulates the urge to push.

But if you have epidural anaesthesia numbing the pelvic nerves, the urge to push is weaker, or absent altogether. That's why women with an epidural have a greater likelihood of having their baby pulled out by a vacuum extractor (suction) or forceps, and an increased chance of Caesarean for what is erroneously *assumed* to be a baby too big to come out.

TAKING THE EDGE OFF: THE REBOUND EFFECT AND DRUG DEPENDENCY

Even though drugs initially ease pain, when the analgesia or anaesthesia wears off, the pain re-experienced will be (suddenly) greater and more difficult to manage than before. This is because when the drugs were first administered, natural endorphins were, still present, easing the pain somewhat.

However, analgesics and anaesthetics send a message to the brain that it no longer needs to produce endorphins. So when the pain medication wears off, there are no endorphins available to buffer the

In 1847, in Edinburgh, "a physician named James Simpson first administered chloroform to a woman who had previously given birth to a still-born child after a three-day labour. When the woman awoke, Simpson had difficulty convincing her that labour was over and that the child before her was really her own.

Simpson was so delighted with the results that he began using chloroform in every labour he attended."[1]

– SHARRON HANNON
CHILDBIRTH: A SOURCE BOOK

intensity of the returning pain. Once a mother accepts drugs "to take the edge off" (especially in early labour), it is difficult to move away from dependency on drugs for pain relief during the rest of labour.

WHOSE PAIN IS IT ANYWAY?

Fathers (and birth companions) often face a special problem with labour pain. Because they love the mother, they may find it unbearable to see her in pain, and may try to rescue her from it. By the same token, a loving wife who sees anguish on her partner's face may acquiesce to drugs just to ease her *partner's* suffering. Medical professionals also have a reflex to relieve pain. All these human reactions can create irresistible pressure towards the otherwise unnecessary use of drugs.

However, as Marsden Wagner, MD, (former Director of Women's and Children's Health for the World Health Organization) observed, "Pain is not evil. It is valuable in birth."[2] Labour pain is manageable with good support and concentration on pain-coping techniques. If the father or nurse advocate drugs during *normal* labour, they need encouragement and guidance from someone with more confidence in birthing-through-pain. Instead of calling for drugs or an epidural, look to your doula for help in maintaining trust, confidence and concentration.

THE RULE OF COMPASSION

In childbirth classes, parents ask me for guidance in knowing *when* to use drugs in labour. Compassion often means relieving pain, so when labour is prolonged, stuck, or induced, the most compassionate response may be the use of drugs or epidural anaesthesia.

In normal childbirth, however, true compassion could mean respecting and supporting a mother's desire and capacity to birth without drugs. If labour is progressing normally, everybody needs to hang tough!

Whether or not a mother eventually uses drugs should not diminish her ability to birth from within. I tell parents that recognizing, accepting, and experiencing whatever is truly needed in their labour *is* birthing from within.

"I figured that birth belonged in the hands of the professionals. So, when the day came, I was hospitalized for the first time in my life. Labouring among strangers and machines, I felt desperate, lonely, and frightened; and I accepted a drug for pain when all I really wanted was help."[3]

– CHRISTINE HALE
"BIRTH AT HOME: AN IMMANENT POWER"
MOTHERING

HOW WILL YOU KNOW LABOUR IS PROGRESSING NORMALLY?

There are many patterns to normal labour; some are strong and fast, like a runaway train, while others progress slowly but steadily. Labour is considered normal when, after reaching four centimetres, dilation progresses at least one centimetre every hour or two. If there is no change in dilation after two hours of good labour, don't give up. During the next hour or two, try every natural intervention you can think of to intensify contractions (e.g., walking, nipple stimulation, baths, massage, or drinking fruit juice or sports drink). If these efforts don't increase dilation, it's time to consider medical interventions (e.g., breaking the water, an IV to rehydrate, syntocin, analgesics or an epidural).

WHEN YOU'RE ALMOST THERE ... BUT DON'T KNOW IT

Near the end of labour (sometimes referred to as "transition"), many mothers believe they still have a long way to go and lose confidence. This was the case with Miquela, who was labouring at home when she began begging to go to the hospital for drugs. At the time she was progressing normally, and was about six centimetres dilated.

First, her midwife validated how intense the pain was for Miquela. In between contractions she explained to Miquela that hard labour helps awaken and prepare the baby for its entry into this world. Then she made a "contract" with Miquela: "Labour as hard as you can for one hour. If you're not close by then and you still want drugs, we'll go to the hospital and get them."

Miquela recommitted herself to her labour. One hour later she was almost ready to push! She was so encouraged and immersed in the labour that she delivered at home without ever mentioning drugs again.

*

BEWARE OF "LABOUR MATH"

Women in labour often do funny calculations in their head. One mother erroneously figured: "It took me eight hours to [thin her cervix and] get to two centimetres dilation … hmmm, that's four hours per centimetre … which means I have another 32 hours to labour! No way … I just can't do it." Discouraged and tired, she scared herself and asked for an epidural (and got it, instead of encouragement, or correction of her labour math).

*

Sometimes a woman who's had a long first labour, panics at the intensity of pain during a faster second labour because she assumes it will take as long as her first one. If she begins to think, "Oh God, I can't take this kind of pain for another 18 hours!" she may beg for drugs. What she really needs is to be told that the pain and intensity will be over *sooner* this time because she's dilating faster (which accounts for the more intense pain).

*

Another hurdle during the home stretch for some mothers may involve a rapid increase in the speed of dilation. A mother might be checked and found to be five centimetres and a little while later start screaming for drugs—because she has suddenly dilated another three centimetres! Before taking any drugs or an epidural have your cervix re-examined (even if it's just been ten minutes). If rapid progress is the cause of your intensified pain, keep going!

*

Most women, when told how imminent the birth is and that they *can* do it (and that they *are* doing it), find the stamina and determination to birth without drugs. That accomplishment generates a special kind of self-confidence they draw on during other difficult times in their lives.

WHEN DRUGS AND EPIDURALS CAN HELP

> "Did the pain techniques work for you?"
>
> "Yeah, they worked great ... for the first twenty-two hours!
> Then I was just too exhausted to cope any more, I really needed
> a pain-killer to get through the last seven hours."
>
> – CONVERSATION OVERHEARD AT A
> POST-PARTUM REUNION

The birth you are living rarely is the one you fantasized, so be prepared to let go of your fantasy. To give birth in *awareness* does not necessarily mean without drugs; it means to be open to each moment and to do whatever *needs* to be done, wholeheartedly. There are certain kinds of labours where expecting yourself to cope with pain is unnecessary, and even unhelpful.

It may be wise and compassionate for mothers to use drugs or an epidural in the following circumstances:

MATERNAL EXHAUSTION: Labour has lasted as long as 24 hours and the baby's birth is not imminent. An exhausted mother needs to sleep.

FAILURE TO PROGRESS: Dilation has stopped, even though strong, regular contractions have been continuing for more than four hours. In cases where labour is stuck, *and every effort has been made to augment it naturally*, using drugs or an epidural may actually normalize labour (and prevent unnecessary psychological birth trauma). Prolonged stress not only exhausts mothers physically and emotionally, it also elevates adrenalin levels. This increased adrenalin neutralizes oxytocin– thereby weakening contractions and slowing or arresting cervical dilation. At this point, relief from pain allows the mother to get some much-needed rest, and a chance to be re-hydrated if necessary.

SYNTOCIN INDUCTION: Labour is being induced or accelerated by syntocin (a synthetic form of oxytocin). Artificially stimulated contractions tend to be more intense. In addition, a cervix that is "unripe" (i.e., long, thick, firm, closed or dilated little) when labour is induced is likely to dilate slowly, making for a long, painful process. Coping also becomes more difficult and stressful because the mother is confined to bed by an IV and foetal monitor.

In this kind of situation, timely relief from pain lowers adrenalin levels and helps the mother relax deeply. Oxytocin levels may then rise, and if they do, the strong, effective contractions necessary for the baby to be born normally will resume. Be aware, sometimes when a mother is already in an abnormal labour pattern (which is why syntocin was used in the first place), relief provided by the epidural or drugs may not be enough to get labour back on track.

NOTE: Sometimes women with a *ripe* cervix (i.e., a cervix that is soft like overripe fruit, and beginning to thin and dilate) do progress quickly with syntocin, and can deliver without any drugs or epidurals. So, don't assume you need to have an epidural with syntocin induction or augmentation. Wait and see.

CAESAREAN BIRTH: Of course, anaesthesia is part of a Caesarean birth.

UNWANTED SIDE EFFECTS OF DRUGS AND EPIDURALS

"Let me ask you something. When you're at the dentist, would you have a tooth pulled or a cavity filled without being numbed first?"

"Well, no."

"So why would you want to go through labour without drugs or an epidural? Labour hurts a lot more, and for a lot longer, than having a little dental work! You think about it, but there's no reason to suffer nowadays to have a baby."

CONVERSATION BETWEEN AN EXPECTANT MUM AND HER DOCTOR.

*

WHY INDEED?

During dental procedures, nothing important is lost when you numb sensation, nor are there any significant risks involved. For most people (older than five) dental work is not a rite of passage; nor is it an important psychological or social transition in their lives. Comparing the sudden, externally-induced pain of dental work (or other surgical procedures), with the pain of normal labour is a misleading analogy.

A better analogy might be the one our friend, Linda, offered: Women's bodies were intended to birth. When baby teeth fall out naturally, we don't need anaesthesia. As labour pain unfolds and intensifies, your body produces endorphins to ease the pain. When pain is abruptly caused by *external* actions, the body has no mechanism in place to help you cope with it.

> "I sincerely regret the introduction of anaesthetics into midwifery: not because they are not useful and laudable in some cases, but from a conviction that the use of them has become a great abuse, which I believe will become greater until the day, not distant one, shall arrive when mankind, and the profession also, shall have been convinced that the doctors have made a mistake on this point."[4]
>
> – DR. CHARLES MEIGS, 1856
> PROFESSOR OF OBSTETRICS,
> JEFFERSON MEDICAL COLLEGE

CASCADING

An epidural during *normal* labour
is not benign pain relief.
You are also relieved of
being-in-labour and
of your power and autonomy
(both emotional and physical).
Having an epidural means you are
confined to bed because you are
continuously hooked-up to:
the epidural tubing inserted in your back and
connected to a clicking, beeping machine …
an IV connected to
another beeping machine …
an external foetal monitor strapped to your belly
or an internal one screwed into your baby's scalp
and connected to a machine
spewing a cascade of paper
drawing the attention of those in the room
away from you …
and a catheter
inserted into your bladder
because you've lost all control.

*

Most women experience decreased pain with an epidural, but not
complete relief. In fact, one study reported that 15 percent of the
women receiving an epidural got no pain relief.[5] According to
another study (Wuitchik, Bakal, and Lipshitz,) the average reduction
in pain relief following an epidural went from the maximum score of
10 to a 5.[6] When weighing the benefits of an epidural, consider
whether the added stress of being confined to bed and enduring further interventions is worth a few hours of lessened pain *(especially* if
you are near the end of labour).

Thorp et al.'s randomized controlled study (1989) found that 19
percent of women with epidurals had a posterior baby persisting into
second stage compared with four percent of the non-epidural group.[7]
Failure to rotate into the more advantageous "facing down" position
is responsible for increases in Caesarean births and forceps/vacuum
extraction deliveries. This is true even when syntocin is given to
strengthen contractions.

"Today various studies show that between 15 and 25 percent of full-
term, healthy babies born to healthy mothers are spending days or
weeks in intensive care units … Why are they there?

   Mostly as a result of the interventions done on their mothers in
labour, which create symptoms in either the mother or the baby that
lead health workers to believe the baby might have a medical
problem."[8]

EPIDURALS INCREASE THE USE OF OTHER MEDICAL INTERVENTIONS AND THEIR RELATED RISKS FOR MOTHERS *AND* BABIES

> "I wonder if women are told this? Women will go through utter hell if they think it's going to be good for the baby. She may accept all of the risks to her. But tell her about the risks to the baby and you've got something else."

MARSDEN WAGNER, MD

1. Because of the potential for epidural-induced foetal heart rate decelerations, it is necessary to use continuous electronic foetal monitoring. Studies have shown that using continuous electronic foetal monitoring increases the Caesarean rate by 2–3 times (without improving the baby's outcome).[9] A drop in foetal heart rate adds worry and stress to labour, and sometimes is serious enough to warrant foetal scalp-blood sampling.

2. When epidural anaesthesia is introduced, the mother's blood pressure often drops, causing serious foetal distress from decreased oxygen circulation. Intravenous fluids must be administered rapidly to counteract this side effect of epidurals in the mother. While this relieves one problem, it creates others, including excessive swelling in the mother's feet, legs and breasts. When the breasts are engorged, the nipple is flattened. This makes it difficult, and sometimes impossible, for the newborn to latch on.

3. Epidural anaesthesia also numbs the bladder, eliminating the sensations which signal the need to urinate. At the same time, huge amounts of IV fluids are flowing into the mother to counteract the anticipated drop in blood pressure. So to prevent bladder distention, a URINARY CATHETER is needed until the epidural wears off. Catheterization brings an added risk of bladder infection, which would then require antibiotic treatment. Studies also show there is a 700 percent increase in urinary incontinence three months after an epidural. Even a year later, incontinence remains 200 percent higher than in non-epidural mums.[10]

4. As explained earlier, epidurals disturb the natural feedback system that stimulates and maintains good, strong labour. If

labour progress slows down or stops altogether, uterine contractions can be artificially stimulated with SYNTOCIN through the IV. Syntocin, even when carefully administered through an electronic "pump," can cause unnaturally strong and prolonged contractions. Such contractions decrease the oxygen supply to the baby causing foetal distress.

This risk requires continuous electronic foetal and uterine monitoring. Unfortunately, continuous electronic foetal monitoring (regardless of why it is being used) increases Caesarean births.

5. One study (Murray, et al, 1981) found that the time it takes to push a baby out is longer for mothers either with an epidural (100.4 minutes) or with syntocin and an epidural (83.8 minutes) compared with unmedicated mothers (47.7 minutes).'[11]

As described elsewhere in this chapter, epidurals interfere with the urge to push, the effectiveness of pushing, the rotation of the baby's head into the most favourable position and the mother's physical capacity to choose her most effective birthing position. That's why with an epidural there is a five-times greater likelihood that FORCEPS OR VACUUM EXTRACTION will be used to pull the baby out.[12] Another study found forceps were used in 60 percent of mothers with epidurals, and 80 percent in mothers with syntocin and epidurals, *but there were no forcep deliveries in the unmedicated group.*

6. THE INCIDENCE OF DEEP VAGINAL TEARS THAT EXTEND INTO THE RECTUM is three times greater with an epidural (because of the related increase of episiotomy and the use of forceps).[13] Deep tears are painful and take longer to heal, and may later cause faecal incontinence, and chronic pain during sex.

7. Studies have shown an INCREASE IN CAESAREAN BIRTH RATE. Thorp, et al. found a Caesarean rate of 17 percent in its epidural group and only 2 percent in the non-epidural group, even though the mothers in the two groups were essentially equivalent before the epidural was administered.[14]

Thorp, et al, (1993) reported that the earlier an epidural is begun, the greater likelihood of Caesarean: They reported a 50% increase in Caesarean birth rate when an epidural was started at 2 cm; 33% at 3 cm; and 26% at 4 cm.[15]

The increased Caesarean rate can be attributed to the following epidural-induced factors:

- Foetal distress brought on by a drop in mother's blood pressure, decreasing placental blood flow;
- Weakening, slowing or stopping of uterine contractions;
- Abnormal position of the baby's head, resulting from a failure to rotate and descend normally during second stage because the epidural has numbed and relaxed pelvic floor muscles (and interrupted the feedback loop);
- Decreased pelvic diameter when the mother is forced to lie on her back.

8. Epidural Fever. The hard work of normal labour raises the mother's temperature slightly, which causes no problems. Epidural "fever," although medically benign, must be treated more seriously.

   The incidence of epidural fever is disturbing. Among epidural-mothers, one in four will develop an epidural fever after four hours, and almost half after eight hours.

   Just two to three hours after an epidural is started, the mother's temperature begins to rise approximately 0.1°C per hour,[16] and 1.0°C (1.8°F) every seven hours.[17,18]

   Fusi, et al (1989) observed that, "The rise in temperature in most women with epidural did not result from an infective process, but from their inability to dissipate the heat generated in the process of labour."[19] They went on to postulate that:

> this inability stemmed from the paralysis of the lumbosacral autonomic nerves which not only produced changes in blood pressure, but also prevented sweating. Since in conditions of heat stress up to 80 percent of body heat production is removed by evaporation of sweat, loss of sweating over the lower half of the body will inevitably cause a positive heat balance with a resulting rise in core body temperature.
>
> … Epidural block therefore seems … to create an imbalance between the heat producing and heat dissipating mechanisms, causing a fever even in the absence of vaginal, uterine or urinary bacterial infection.[20]

However, because infection can have serious consequences for both mother and baby, once a fever develops aggressive medical management must be undertaken.

A rise in the mother's temperature (from whatever cause) may result in a rise in the foetus' as well, causing dramatically increased heart rate and possible metabolic deterioration. Medical management of this condition includes intravenous antibiotic therapy, and speeding up labour with syntocin, forceps, vacuum extraction or Caesarean.

Infection in newborn babies is extremely serious and must be treated immediately. Neonatal intensive care nurses I interviewed explained that "some babies born to mothers with fevers in labour, depending on the circumstances, get septic workups. But all babies born with an elevated temperature are put in intensive care nursery for a septic workup."

What does a septic workup involve? Blood is drawn from the baby at least once (and as often as every few hours), and sometimes a spinal tap is performed. A spinal tap entails inserting a needle into the outer covering of the spinal cord in order to sample the fluid that bathes the spinal cord. The fluid is cultured in a lab to see whether an infection is present.

Infection in a newborn can be life-threatening. So, even before results have come back from blood work or spinal taps to show whether an infection is actually present, antibiotics and treatment must begin. At the very least this situation creates tremendous stress and worry, an emotionally painful separation from the baby, and interference with breastfeeding.

All this pain, anxiety and expense for what is usually found to be a benign epidural fever (which requires no treatment). Yet, the workup must be done to avoid missing the timely diagnosis and treatment of an actual infection.

9. It is a popular myth that epidural medication doesn't get to the baby. Epidural anaesthetics *do* cross the placental barrier. Anaesthetic levels in the baby's blood have been found to be as high as one-third of maternal blood levels.[21,22] As a result, compared to the unmedicated babies, babies in the epidural or syntocin-epidural groups showed "drugged behaviour" (e.g., trembling, irritability, and immature motor activity) on the first day, with behavioural recovery by the *fifth day*. It takes 48 hours

for a newborn to eliminate the epidural anaesthetic from its system.[22]

When syntocin was used with the epidural, there was an even greater depression of motor activity. Babies were more tense, hypertonic, and displayed depressed reflexes.

Murray, et al, discovered that *a month after birth*, unmedicated mothers reported their babies to be more sociable, rewarding, and easy to care for than did the epidural mothers. In addition, the unmedicated mothers were more responsive to their babies' cries than mothers who had epidural anaesthesia in labour.

The early days of the mother-baby relationship may impact bonding and the future of that relationship. The baby's behaviour makes a powerful first impression. When in the first month, babies appear "disorganized" (which means they are more irritable, withdrawn, look away and suckle less) mothers are more likely to perceive them as difficult babies. That impression can affect the mother, unconsciously, in ways that shape her behaviour toward her newborn, which over time, will shape the baby's personality and consequently the mother-baby relationship.[23]

SO, IF YOUR DOCTOR TELLS YOU "EPIDURALS ARE A WOMAN'S BEST FRIEND," DON'T BELIEVE IT!

*

A WORD ABOUT WALKING EPIDURALS

"Walking epidurals—that is a joke. Don't take it seriously."

PENNY SIMKIN, P.T.
AUTHOR OF *THE BIRTH PARTNER*

The walking epidural is also referred to as narcotic analgesia or narcotic epidural. The anaesthesiologist uses a mixture of narcotic and local anaesthetic (bupivacaine). "Depending on the proportion of narcotic to anaesthetic, the concentration of anaesthetic, and the mother's individual sensory and motor response, she may be able to sit in a chair or even walk after receiving this epidural."[24]

In a lecture at the Midwifery Today Conference (1996) Penny Simkin explained that 55 percent of mothers with a "walking epidural" lose their proprioceptor sense and cannot walk. This means when they put their foot down, they don't know where it is. So, unless someone else moves their feet for them, and two people hold them up, they can't walk.[25]

*

"Walking epidurals?!
That's a misnomer. First of all there's nowhere to walk to—you're attached to a monitor, IV pole, and catheter. Anyway, by the time many mothers get an epidural, they're exhausted and fall into a deep sleep."

ANASTASIA OTT, R.N.,
LABOUR AND DELIVERY NURSE

SYNTOCIN: GOOD NEWS/BAD NEWS

"Oxytocin [syntocin] has done more to raise the living standards of medical-malpractice attorneys than any other drug on the market."

OVERHEARD BY DORIS HAIRE
HEAD OF NIH DEPARTMENT OF ENDOCRINOLOGY,
AT THE NEW YORK STATE TRIAL LAWYERS ASSOCIATION CONFERENCE

Syntocin is synthetic oxytocin that works by stimulating the smooth muscles of the uterus and blood vessels. Syntocin stimulates, or increases the strength of, uterine contractions.

GOOD NEWS:

There are certain obstetrical situations where the benefits of syntocin outweigh the risks. For example, syntocin can get a stuck labour moving again. Completely exhausted mothers may need a syntocin-boost to finish labour. Syntocin can also jump-start labour in overdue mothers (42 weeks gestation).

Syntocin may also be useful when the water has broken and contractions are weak or haven't started (depending on the situation, 12–24 hours may elapse before syntocin augmentation is considered). The danger of infection may be avoided because syntocin helps the baby get born in a timely manner.

BAD NEWS:

In the hope you'll feel informed but not fearful, we've listed possible complications involved with the use of syntocin:

MATERNAL:

- Hyperstimulation of the uterus resulting in prolonged (tetanic) contractions, which can cause:

  > Premature separation of the placenta (abruptio placenta)
  > Uterine rupture resulting in emergency Caesarean birth or death
  > Decreased oxygen to the baby (because of reduced uterine blood flow)
  > Rapid labour and delivery resulting in cervical or perineal lacerations, pelvic haematoma, and trauma to the newborn

- Water intoxication (because syntocin is an anti-diuretic) leading to an irregular heart beat, hypotension, nausea and vomiting, excessive swelling, and difficulty nursing.

FOETAL OR NEWBORN:

- Tetanic contractions cause decreased oxygen supply to the foetus, resulting in foetal heart rate decelerations.
- Newborn jaundice
- Decreased platelet aggregation (clotting capacity)

Because the risk of complications associated with syntocin is significant, it's worthwhile exploring non-drug alternatives to augmenting or stimulating labour (see p. 332).

*

If syntocin is being suggested to induce labour, first find out whether your cervix is "ripe." Syntocin dilates a ripe cervix, it does not "ripen" the cervix.

If labour is progressing too slowly or is stuck, before agreeing to syntocin augmentation, consider the following:

- **Is my environment part of my problem?**
  Do you need more privacy? Is someone present making you self-conscious? Is the room dark, warm, and quiet?
- **Do I need to be rehydrated?**
  Force fluids, an IV, anti-emetics (if vomiting is a problem).
- **Is weakness and exhaustion my real problem?**
  Take a sleeping pill or narcotic to help you get some rest. A warm lavender bath and massage may be the soothing boost you need. (Eventually, you may benefit from an epidural.)
- **Are there other more natural ways to stimulate labour?**
  Nipple stimulation, love-making (if your water has not broken), enema or castor oil cocktail (2 oz of castor oil mixed well in 2 oz orange juice) to stimulate intestinal activity which sometimes triggers uterine contractions), or herbs (Black Cohash, Blue Cohash).
- **What can my midwife or doctor do to stimulate labour before using syntocin?**
  Strip membranes, artificially rupture the water, apply prostaglandin gel on the cervix, and carefully re-assess physical factors which may be keeping the labour from progressing. Ask them about these options.

MATERNAL WISDOM CAN COME FROM THE UNEXPECTED

Whitney, a 36-year-old first-time mum and successful computer business executive, was a model of determination and confidence throughout her healthy pregnancy and childbirth classes. Her expectation and intention was to birth normally, without drugs.

But in the birth-world parents often must face the unexpected. Whitney's labour was gruelling and prolonged. After 27 hours of contractions, she was discouraged to learn she had only dilated to 1 centimetre. She had tried to enhance her labour in every natural way possible, including herbs, acupuncture, baths and massage, all to no avail.

Exhausted and dehydrated, Whitney was encouraged by her support team to accept an epidural in the hope that relief from unproductive pain would allow her to get much-needed rest. While considering this offer, Whitney cried and grieved the loss of her image of giving birth.

She persisted in labouring four more hours. When the doctor told her she was only 2 centimetres dilated, Whitney realized her body was not going to give birth without additional help. She accepted the epidural, and rested.

Even with the aid of an epidural and syntocin, labour dragged on another 16 hours before her daughter was born! Later, she shared with her postpartum group a profound insight about herself:

> I've always accomplished what I set out to do. I've been successful in sports and my profession. I trusted my body, and my ability to birth naturally.
>
> So, when I was told I was not making progress, I just could not believe it. I was physically and emotionally spent—I had nothing left to draw on. Facing the need to have an epidural was a crisis for me.
>
> I needed the loving support and acceptance from my birth partner and friends to know I was doing the right thing, and that I was not weak or giving up easily. They told me how strong I had been, and cried with me. [Whitney cried in the group as she recounted that touching moment.]
>
> Later, I realized that all my life I had been in control. Whenever I set my mind to do something, I made it happen. I thought giving birth and mothering would be the same way. Losing control of my labour and having the epidural was a gift because it made me realize that as a mother I could not have the kind of control I was used to in other areas of my life. I'm learning that though I might have ideas about my baby and mothering, I can't always control what happens. And I'm still able to be a good mother.

A WORD OF ENCOURAGEMENT

If you're progressing and you've been told you only have a few more hours to go in labour—JUST DO IT—without drugs or epidural. Use the techniques in this book or anything else that you can call on. You can do it—it's manageable. Do it for your health and the health of your baby.

If labour is abnormal and the benefits of drugs or anaesthesia outweigh their risks, welcome them. Accept that you did the best that you could, and stay present and involved in your birth in every way you can. Remember, an epidural doesn't need to stop you from birthing from within.

SECTION VII

Gestating Parenthood

Chapter 40

Gestating Motherhood

> While a baby is gestating so is motherhood. When a baby is
> born, so are its mother and father "born."

Given adequate nutrition, a foetus grows without effort from its parents. However, the development of your parent-identity is not
necessarily an automatic process of nature. If you want to help this
happen, you'll have to play an active part.

Your successful evolution to parenthood depends largely on your
accommodation to the vast changes which are unfolding beyond
your control. Learning to accept loss of control is an integral part of
both birth and motherhood/fatherhood.

For example, beginning in pregnancy, you gradually will have less
and less control over your emotions, bodily functions or sleep. In
labour (especially without drugs) you will be forced to surrender the
masks of your ego. All of these changes remind you that your life style
and self are being irrevocably transformed.

"I feel like I'm being
held in the womb of
the Great Mother. My
baby isn't the only
one gestating, it feels
like I'm gestating too,
for motherhood. In
the picture, I've given
birth and I'm holding
my baby."
VANESSA

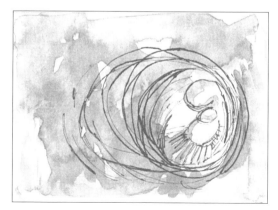

Accompanying the birth of your new life is the "death" of your old one. A healthy gestation includes acknowledging what you are giving up (at least for a while): sleep, spontaneously going to a movie, party, or away for the weekend, income, plans for career or education, and the marital relationship as you've known it.

Most new parents are caught off guard by the unexpected, almost painful, intensity of love and attachment to their newborn baby. This intensity introduces a new vulnerability to life which upsets your emotional equilibrium. The other side of loving your wonderful, yet helpless, infant is the overwhelming fear of losing your baby. This terror dwells in the depths of your new-parent consciousness. This dynamic balance of love and fear, and the protective and nurturant behaviours it generates, is the essence of parenthood.

WHO WILL ASSIST YOUR "BIRTH" AS PARENTS?

The great life passages from maidenhood to motherhood, from being a couple to being parents, are virtually overlooked by health professionals. (As you've already noticed, prenatal care and childbirth classes emphasize physical and medical considerations.) Yet the outcome of this less visible gestational process will determine the health of your family for years to come.

Because modern obstetric training and responsibility focuses on body care, it's unrealistic, if not unfair, to expect medical people to guide you through this emotional-psychological transition. Accept that it is your responsibility to search out and connect with helpful people and experiences. Guidance and support through the transition of *parenthood* falls more naturally to family, friendship, spirituality and, at times, therapy.

WHAT DOES A HEALTHY "NEWBORN" MOTHER OR FATHER LOOK LIKE?

A paediatrician knows what a healthy newborn baby looks like. But what does a heathy newborn parent look like?

Although values differ across cultures and time, we've identified some qualities that may be indicators of a healthy new parent in our culture:

- Deeply rooted sense of protectiveness
- Acceptance of the loss of control (over one's life, time, and emotions) while developing a deeper sense of humour and absurdity
- Acceptance of responsibility for the parts of your child's development which you can control (e.g., discipline)
- Willingness to be self-sacrificing
- Understanding interdependence (People sometimes think of immaturity as being too dependent. Another kind of immaturity is not being able to ask for help.)
- Patience, flexibility and creativity
- Awareness of how your own childhood affects your parenting
- Acceptance of your changed physical-social identities

WHAT TO DO:

1. On your own or in a group ... Draw/Write/Discuss what your transition to parenthood looks like.
2. Discuss with friends or a childbirth class your reactions to this chapter and the following questions:
   - How did you see yourself as an individual/couple before your pregnancy?
   - How do you envision yourself as a new parent with your baby?
   - How do you imagine your partner as a parent?
   - What image of yourself as parent makes you most anxious?
   - How do you want your baby to see you? What would you want your baby to say about you if he/she could chat with other babies at his/her first birthday party?

PREMATURE PARENTHOOD

PREMATURE (pre * ma * turé) [L. *prematurus; prae*, before, and *maturus*, ripe] happening, arriving, coming to pass unexpectedly early, too early.

While a baby born prematurely can survive its mis-timed arrival through the intensive, miraculous support of medical technology, mothers and fathers suffering from *premature parenthood* are often misunderstood and left to fend for themselves.

Premature parents are those who conceive before they or their relationship are psychologically, socially, or financially ready. The baby is not necessarily unwanted or even unplanned.

FACTORS ASSOCIATED WITH PREMATURE PARENTHOOD:

- Unfinished education
- Unresolved issues with parents
- Inadequate financial resources
- Unfulfilled wanderlust
- A partnership still in its early, non-solidified stages (or no partner at all)
- Unreadiness of the extended family to help (e.g., premature grandparenthood).

COMPLICATIONS OF PREMATURE PARENTHOOD

For some, premature parenthood may wind up being a temporary period of frustration. But for others, it is potentially serious, and may have a long-term, damaging effect on their family's well-being.

Premature parents are at risk to develop any of the following:

- Resentment
- Depression
- Anger
- Guilt
- Over-protectiveness
- Negligence
- Free-floating anxiety
- Lack of confidence
- Damaged self-esteem
- Isolation
- Shame
- Marital discord or separation
- Child neglect or abuse

Sometimes when expectant parents are detoured from their *personal* aspirations, there is an over-eagerness to get their lives back on track. This may result in high expectations of their baby, their partner and themselves, thereby creating an undercurrent of tension, resentment and blame in the family.

Caring for a new baby in the absence of adequate personal/marital resources can harm a family by draining physical and emotional energy away from the marriage. The couple may experience isolation, stagnation, or even the withering of what previously had been a satisfactory relationship.

When a baby arrives before the parents are ready, the ability to parent skillfully, with patience and understanding, is also undermined. When premature parents are not comfortable with their own emotions (especially neediness, anger, and sadness) they communicate judgement, resentment and rejection of their infant/child's normal emotions and behaviour. This leads to negative mother-child or father-child interactions, erosion of self esteem, and increasingly painful, conflicted family relationships.

WHAT'S A PREMATURE PARENT TO DO?

These complex issues can't be resolved without effort, and frequently professional guidance is necessary. The following may be helpful:

- Individual or marital therapy during pregnancy
- Postpartum therapy
- Postpartum support groups
- Read books or take a class on parenting skills
- Take a Baby-Proofing Your Marriage Workshop or a Marriage Enrichment Weekend

Chapter 41

Baby-Proofing Your Marriage

Images of poisoned or injured babies activate you to baby-proof your home. But what about baby-proofing your marriage?

Successful postpartum adjustment comes from awareness, and realistic preparation, not blissful fantasizing. Our Baby-proofing and Postpartum Connections classes warn couples that beautiful images of bonded, loving, joyful new families can distract them from learning the skills they need to navigate the rough waters of new parenthood. This chapter contains a sampling of what we talk about with couples in our postpartum groups.

In their excellent book, *The Transition to Parenthood: How A First Child Changes a Marriage* (1994), researchers Jay Belsky and John Kelly reported that previous research indicated "there was only one major form of marital change among new parents—decline." But what they found in their own research surprised them: "Our data [on 250 couples] indicated that a marriage can change in one of four ways, and in each case the direction of change is determined by the couple's ability to overcome the polarizing effects of the transition."[1]

In order to study the impact of the transition from couplehood to parenthood, couples were followed from the third trimester of pregnancy to the child's third birthday. Belsky and Kelly found couples fell into one of four categories: Severe Decliners (12%); Moderate Decliners (39%); No Change (30%); and Improvers (19%).[2]

WHAT WERE THE "IMPROVERS" DOING?

Improvers were described as those whom "the process of overcoming transition-time, marital gaps and divisions brought … closer together."

Only 19 percent of the couples studied actually achieved what all of us hope our baby's arrival will bring. Some of the characteristics that Belsky and Kelly proposed as "most important in facilitating a husband's and wife's smooth passage through the transition included the ability to surrender individual goals and needs and work together as a team, … to merge their individual selves into a larger Us, and to resolve differences about division of household chores and work—in a mutually satisfactory manner."

The husbands and wives in the study agreed that "this is the major stress of the transition … and while they expected the baby to create a lot more work, that expectation did not prepare them for what they actually encountered. One of the [study] mothers compared the difference to 'watching a tornado on TV and having one actually blow the roof off your house.'"[3]

SURVIVAL HINTS:

- Lower your housekeeping standards (Throw away your white gloves!).
- Recognize that baby care and household chores can't be divided 50–50; at any given moment one parent inevitably will be doing more in one area while the other does more in another. Try not to keep score.
- Consider hiring a housekeeper (if you can afford it) until you adjust to the chaos.
- Fight constructively. In our classes and counselling, time is spent discussing the differences between constructive versus destructive conflict. Couples learn ground rules for fighting, how to follow up on issues raised during a fight (once tempers have cooled), and how to finish a fight so bad feelings don't go on endlessly.
- Realize that however good a marriage becomes postbaby, it will not be good in the *same way* it was prebaby.
- Keep in mind whether your communication is nurturing or harming the marriage.[4]

TRY PREDICTING YOUR POSTBABY SQUABBLES.

ZEN DUST, ZEN SWEEP

"It's a small activity, sweeping, but it leaves the floor calmer, and livelier at the same time. Awakened ...

There is something humbling and balance-bringing about housework, something humble about washing a rock. In the doing of such work primal memories are awakened, memories to do with the human-shelter-world arrangement ...

It seems as if housework is something a lot of people would rather not do—some kind of punishment for living in the material world ...

It is not necessary to be victimized by the demands of the home. Along with family, work, play, spiritual pursuits, all the spheres of involvement in life, the house-home too is a primary presence ... it is the foundation, the source, and the center from which one departs and to which one returns. It forms the visible encircling image of family union ...

It is just consciousness—attitude—that transforms drudgery into ritual ... The way is simple. Approach your task respectfully. Start small. Hold back expectation. Give time, allow ritual to emerge, enjoy the play of it, focus on the process, the act, the object. Dust absolutely; be a virtuoso on the broom. Washing a rock, one finds rocklike presence within. Clean cobwebs from your soul!"

— DOMINIQUE LEIGH
"ZEN DUST, ZEN SWEEP"
MOTHER MAGAZINE[6]

WHAT DIVIDES NEW PARENTS

Even Improvers said they were surprised by how many more disagreements they had after the baby arrived. (Before reading on, imagine five things you and your partner are most likely to argue about postbaby.)

According to Belsky and Kelly's research, "new parents disagree about many things, but when they fight they usually fight about one of five things:

- Division of labour
- Money
- Work
- Their relationship (which one of them is to blame for the postpartum disconnection, loneliness, and stress)
- Social life (are we getting out enough?)

"These five issues are so big, important, and all pervasive they might be said to constitute the raw material of marital change during the transition. Quite simply, couples who manage to resolve these issues in a mutually satisfactory way become happier with their marriage, whereas those who do not become unhappier."[5]

ISSUE NUMBER SIX: IN-LAWS

Our clinical experience makes it impossible not to include a huge issue couples struggle with postpartum: in-laws. The addition of a baby to a couple's relationship puts new urgency into the question of family boundaries. In-laws now may feel a heightened sense of involvement in what is going on over at "the kids' house." This shared area of interest (the baby) can enrich, reconnect, and heal the relationships between parents and their adult children. But it also can exacerbate on-going tensions around respect, autonomy, and loyalty.

For many young adults marriage initiates a process of differentiation and boundary-setting vis-a-vis their family of origin. But the new family created by the arrival of the baby makes these issues even more salient. Redefining relationships (especially with a loving parent) can be a poignant, even scary rite of passage.

New parents benefit from well-timed advice and assistance.

Unfortunately some in-laws go overboard; overwhelmed and exhausted mums and dads can easily wind up feeling irritated, criticized, or undermined.

Negotiating this awkward transition is accomplished most effectively when the spouse whose family-of-origin is over-involved and/or intrusive takes the leadership role. When the other spouse tries to confront this in-law issue without support from his/her partner, the situation often becomes worse: the original circumstances remain unchanged (or even inflamed), and the spouse who raised the issue now feels betrayed. His/her fear feels confirmed: the primary place in the partner's heart is reserved for the family-of-origin. In counseling, many serious marital problems can be traced back to this heated issue being unresolved, and left to smolder.

A key transition task then is learning to clearly, but graciously, set limits if you feel disrespected or overwhelmed by in-laws. How you resolve this challenge will influence whether you eventually find yourself in a supportive extended family, or embroiled in chronic, bitter arguments.

Are you as new parents prepared to make a commitment to your new family?

Or will painful love and loyalty conflicts involving your families of origin compromise the integrity of your new family?

*

This chapter is intended to be a preview of postpartum issues, not a complete Baby-Proofing guide. In Albuquerque, parents can take our Baby-Proofing workshop or Postpartum Connections classes.

If these specific resources are not available in your area, you can begin your baby-proofing by sitting down and talking with other new parents about their transition. Another possibility, and usually a wise financial investment, is to schedule a few pre-baby planning/counselling sessions with someone familiar with postpartum adjustment issues.

WHAT YOU CAN DO:

WRITE A POSTPARTUM ADJUSTMENT PLAN

1. Without consulting with your partner, each of you write down five issues you anticipate could be a problem in your relationship after your baby is born
2. Share your lists with one another. Listen without interrupting while your partner talks about his or her concerns.
   Try not to be defensive.
3. Brainstorm together; consider (and write down) *all* possible solutions, including far-fetched ones.
4. From your lists, choose one or two solutions that seem most likely to ease each problem.
5. If you were to implement a solution, what would be your first SMALL step? Write it down. When the time comes, Do It!
6. Think of this list as a Postpartum Life Preserver, and keep it visible. Hang it on your bedroom mirror or refrigerator.

*

A new crib and pretty wallpaper
in the nursery are sweet, but
the best gift for your newborn is
Baby-proofing your marriage.

*

Chapter 42

Swaddling The New Parents

When the mother leaves the hut the first time after the birth, she emerges dressed specially, in her hand a staff such as is carried by the elders, followed by the child who cooks for her. Sedately they take their way to the market, where they are greeted with songs such as were sung to the warriors returning from battle.

WACHAGGA OF UGANDA

… Birth was a time of honor for most tribal mothers. A woman in childbirth was treated with the same respect as a man in battle. In fact, in the tribal mind, there was a metaphysical equation between the two acts.

JUDITH GOLDSMITH
CHILDBIRTH WISDOM

In many traditional cultures new mothers and babies rejoin their community, with no fuss or ceremony, within an hour of birth. In others, they are isolated from the rest of the community, bathed, massaged, and pampered for weeks. This allows the mother to integrate her birth experience and adapt to her new status in society, as well as physically recover from the birth. She and the baby then re-enter the group through a welcoming ceremony.

Unfortunately, modern medicalized-birth cultures do not recognize or celebrate new mothers. There is decreasing cultural support to help new couples through the isolation, transitions, and upheavals that follow the birth of their baby. (This is especially true with the breakdown of extended families, and pressure for women to return quickly to the workforce.)

The medical model's six week postpartum exam has become our bleak postpartum transition ritual. The mother is given a physical exam, birth control and clearance to attack her "in-basket" at work. New mothers have confided in me how they long to be ceremonially or publicly recognized by other mothers and friends for what they have accomplished and become. Think about how you might like to be celebrated after your baby is born. You will deserve it!

TRANSITION TIPS

ACKNOWLEDGE WHAT YOU AND YOUR PARTNER HAVE LOST

After the arrival of your baby, there is less sleep, spontaneity, money, and time to be together or pursue individual interests.

Try not to compete with your spouse for who's sacrificed more or who has the greater claim to total exhaustion. Recognize that your partner is under stress, too, and make an effort to practice loving kindness with one another.

GIVE YOURSELF TIME TO REST

Take your phone off the hook; turn on your answering machine. Hang a "Do Not Disturb" sign on your door.

HOLD ON TO YOUR SENSE OF HUMOUR

Laugh at your own frazzled floundering and incompetence. Don't worry about being a "perfect" parent—babies are easily fooled!

SET UP MEALS ON WHEELS

It's nearly impossible for new parents to juggle taking care of a new-born baby, household chores, going to work, shopping *and* getting meals prepared. Yet eating well is essential to producing adequate breastmilk, and for your sense of well-being. So, here's how to organize early postpartum Meals On Wheels:

Before your baby is born, ask someone to contact friends and family to arrange for them to provide a postpartum meal. If you have food allergies, fetishes, or preferences, let your organizer know. There are several strategies for making this happen.

One way is to suggest a frozen meal be a "gift" at a Mother Blessing or Baby Shower.

*

Another approach is to make a Meals on Wheels Calendar marking days 1 through 14. Day 1 will be the first day after the baby's birth. Each "cook" chooses one or two numbers between 1 and 14, and agrees to bring a prepared meal to your home at a designated time on the day that corresponds to her (or his) number.

For example, if Aunt Millie picks number 6, she will bring a meal and dessert on the sixth day after your baby is born. If there are left-overs, freeze them so they can rescue you at a later mealtime.

*

The visiting "meal-angel" can put your prepared meal in the oven, and while it's warming, set the table, and do an errand or a chore for you. Maybe they could prepare a herbal bath, put on some music, and watch your baby while you take a deserved and leisurely break before dinner.

*

By the way, the meal-angel should not plan on staying for dinner—long visits are tiring for new parents.

POSTPARTUM HEALING AND BODY CARE

AFTERPAINS

Afterpains are strong, menstrual-like cramps that occur as your uterus is contracting back into shape. These are to be expected while nursing your second or later babies but are less likely after your first.

Using a heating pad, taking warm baths and practising mindful concentration pain techniques will all help. If your afterpains are severe, it's safe to take paracetamol or ibuprofen while nursing. Afterpains are usually gone after three days.

BLEEDING

Postpartum uterine bleeding (or "lochia") resembles a heavy period the first few days after birth. It is normal to have a gush of blood or pass a few small clots the first day, especially after you've been lying in bed for a few hours or overnight. By the end of the first week, the flow changes from a red, moderate flow to a watery pink discharge, followed by brown-spotting, until it ceases altogether (two to six weeks after birth).

UTERINE INVOLUTION (RETURNING TO NORMAL SIZE)

Immediately after your placenta is delivered, your uterus contracts down to the size of a grapefruit, to keep you from bleeding. (You can reach down and feel it through your abdomen, just above your pubic bone.) A few hours later, it will relax a little and rise upwards until the top of it reaches the level of your belly button.

Each day afterwards, the uterine muscle contracts and shrinks back downward at a rate of one fingerbreadth a day. By two weeks, and sometimes sooner, the uterus is below the pubic bone and can no longer be felt from the abdomen. While this is happening, the uterine lining (where the placenta was attached) is regenerating.

Women who feel great after giving birth run the risk of doing too much too soon. Others do too much because they don't have enough help or don't understand the need for rest. In early postpartum, when the uterus is still in contact with the abdominal muscles, activity can slow down uterine involution and increase bleeding.

To prevent postpartum haemorrhage and infection, our grand-mothers were kept on bed- or house-rest for ten days after birth. Here's what you should do until your bleeding stops:

- Don't lift anything heavier than your baby (laundry, groceries, or a toddler).
- Remain under "house arrest"—don't drive or do unnecessary errands. Getting in and out of a car, carrying groceries or a baby carrier all use abdominal muscles and can put a strain on your uterus during this time of recovery.
- Avoid vigourous exercising (e.g., aerobics, swimming, biking, running or weight lifting).
- Abstain from sexual intercourse. (Other ways of being intimate and close don't need to be neglected.)

ABNORMAL BLEEDING

If you inadvertently do too much, you might start bleeding heavier or bright red again. Take this as a warning sign to slow down. If you don't have a fever, abdominal pain or foul-smelling lochia, go to bed with your baby and a good novel or stack of videos for 24 hours. Stay put, nurse your baby, eat and drink well. The bleeding should slow down or stop.

Bleeding (lochia) should be considered abnormal when:

- Your flow is heavy and bright red, and saturates a pad in two hours or less (instead of four to six hours);
- Your flow has increased or become bright red—after it was pink or just spotting, and doesn't slow down with rest;
- You are cramping and passing clots after the first day or two;
- The lochia is foul-smelling, and you have a temperature over 100.4°, abdominal pain and general malaise.

In any of these circumstances, call your midwife or doctor immediately. Abnormal bleeding could be caused by retained placenta or membranes and/or uterine infection. These conditions are serious and need medical attention.

PERINEAL CARE

Even if you don't tear or get an episiotomy, your bottom probably will be a little sore the first few days or weeks after giving birth. If you needed stitches, they will be absorbed by your body in a week or two.

Here's what you can do to speed healing:

FROZEN PADS

Immediately after birth, and for the first 24 hours, ice packs or frozen kotex pads reduce perineal and haemorrhoidal swelling and pain.

Instead of lumpy, hard ice packs, some women prefer kotex or washcloths folded in thirds, saturated with sitz bath herbs, and frozen. These are softer and absorb blood better.

TAKE SOOTHING WARM HERBAL SITZ BATHS

Make up, or buy pre-packaged herbal sitz bath mixture from a herb store. (It's best to do this before birth so you have it ready.)

MEET YOUR HERBAL FRIENDS:

- Comfrey—builds new cells rapidly which speeds healing, softens skin and soothes wounds; decreases itching and pain
- Rosemary—a mild antiseptic
- Yarrow—astringent and antibacterial
- Marshmallow root—soothes inflamed, swollen tissues
- UVA URSI—antibiotic properties
- Goldenseal—antibiotic properties
- MYRRH—helps keep herbs fresh

MAKE A SITZ BATH HERBAL INFUSION (TEA):

Simmer 1–2 ounces of herb blend per four–eight cups of water for 20 to 30 minutes. Strain the herbs and pour 2 cups of the infusion into your sitz bath. Save the rest in a jar for later.

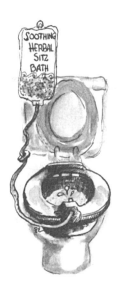

For a week to ten days, take a daily 20-minute, warm sitz bath to help keep the perineal area clean and increase circulation (which speeds healing). Sitz baths can be taken either in a shallow bath which concentrates the herb, or by sitting in a disposable, plastic sitz bath that fits in your toilet. The disposable sitz bath comes with a litre bag and attached tubing. You can fill the bag with herbal infusion and then gently spray your stitches clean.

HONEY ON YOUR PAD

Apply raw honey to pad or a frozen washcloth. Honey is a natural astringent, is soothing and reduces the likelihood of infection.

SUNLIGHT

If possible, expose your bottom to sunlight or air daily. (A wound always covered with a pad is an excellent environment for breeding bacteria.)

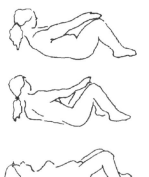

STRENGTHENING ABDOMINAL MUSCLE TONE

Begin abdominal exercises three days to a week postpartum. They take just a few minutes so make them a regular part of your day. More tone will be restored if you exercise the first six weeks postpartum than if you begin these exercises later. Ask your childbirth teacher, midwife or health club instructor for specific instructions.

LOVEMAKING

Lovemaking should not be resumed before bleeding has completely stopped, and any stitches are absorbed (about three to four weeks postpartum).

KEGELS: VAGINAL TONING EXERCISES

Your pelvic floor is a strong sling of muscles attached to your pubic bone and coccyx. Some of these muscles form a figure-eight around your vagina and urethra, others form a sphincter around your anus. You become aware of these muscles when you squeeze or relax them to stop or start urinating. If you can't control the flow of urine, it means your pelvic floor muscles are weak.

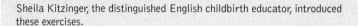

Sheila Kitzinger, the distinguished English childbirth educator, introduced these exercises.

RESTORING VAGINAL TONE

Begin doing your Kegel exercises about the third day postpartum. Your muscle tone will be weak after giving birth, if you can feel it at all! Don't despair—just Kegel every day. At first, Kegel while urinating—see if you can stop and start your stream.

Exercising or toning the vaginal muscles during *pregnancy* increases perineal elasticity, thereby allowing it to stretch more easily over the baby's head in birth.

Kegel exercises prevent or minimize the relaxation of your pelvic floor after birth, whch helps avoid certain inconveniences such as involuntary urination when you sneeze or cough. If that doesn't motivate you, how about this? Strong vaginal muscles improve your sex life by increasing the pleasurable sensations during lovemaking and by strengthening orgasm.

Regardless of how much other exercise you get, *only* Kegel exercises tone your vaginal/perineal muscles. Try one of the Kegel visualizations below:

THE ELEVATOR KEGEL

Imagine pulling the "sling" between your pubic and coccyx bones upward—like an elevator, pulling it up to the first floor, second floor, third floor ... squeezing steadily for five to six seconds. Then, releasing slowly, go down to the second floor, first floor, then open the "door." Rest four to five seconds. Repeat ten times.

KANGAROO KEGELS

If elevators are too mechanical for you, try Kangaroo Kegels. Pretend you are a kangaroo. Slowly lift your great tail into the air, hold it up for five to six seconds. Then, lower it slowly to the ground—without making any dust. Repeat ten times.

*

To achieve a daily total of 100 to 200 Kegels, do 10 to 20 sets throughout your day. It'll be easier for you to remember to do your Kegels if you associate them with an activity you are likely to perform ten times a day (e.g., stopping at a red light, answering the telephone, changing nappies). Put a Kegel reminder sticker on the rear view mirror, telephone, or above the baby's changing table.

Even then, many women, exhausted and preoccupied with the full time care of their new baby, are not interested in sexual intimacy. When the baby is finally asleep, they are desperate to get some things done, or may collapse into sleep themselves.

Because nursing lowers oestrogen levels, nursing mothers often experience vaginal dryness. When you do make love, use oil or a water-soluble jelly to lubricate the vagina. Some women who are extremely dry and tender will find relief with a hormonal cream which can be prescribed by a doctor or nurse-midwife.

Oxytocin is released during lovemaking, labour, and nursing. So, during orgasm postpartum, the release of oxytocin may also stimulate the let-down reflex causing your breasts to leak. Don't worry, there will still be enough milk for your baby.

There is a similarity between labour and lovemaking: the breathing pattern, primal noises, contracting of the uterus (although much milder in lovemaking)—all are induced by oxytocin and involve a sexual release. So, for some mothers, making love soon after giving birth blurs with the memory of being in labour. This unexpected experience can be confusing and upsetting, but is actually quite common. Nothing needs to be done about it. In time, you will not associate lovemaking with labour.

BIRTH CONTROL

If you are bottlefeeding, you can expect to ovulate two to six weeks after delivery.

However, breastfeeding women can begin ovulating at any time. This is especially true if breastfeeding-on-demand has been interrupted for any reason, even one time (e.g., the baby or mother being sick; needing to supplement feeding with a bottle when returning to work or taking a much-needed break with her partner).

Unless a breastfeeding mother is checking for ovulation daily, she may not realize it happened until she has a period (two weeks later)—or has signs of pregnancy. So if you're not wanting to get pregnant during this time, it is best to use birth control. Discuss your options with your doctor or midwife.

BREASTFEEDING

Breastfeeding is such a complex subject, that the important details are beyond the scope of this book. For an in-depth presentation of practical information in a wonderfully illustrated book, we recommend *Bestfeeding* by Mary Renfrew, et al. (1990).

Here's just a nipple-full of information. Some of the advantages of breastfeeding include:

BREAST MILK IS CUSTOM-MADE FOR EVERY BABY

Breast milk is precisely designed to meet the needs of the developing brain and body of a baby. In fact, it is so precisely fitted to a baby's needs that the composition of the mother's milk actually changes in direct response to the needs of her baby. No one yet knows exactly how this happens. A prematurely born baby receives breast milk of a very different composition—in terms of the protein and fat content and trace nutrients—than a full-term baby, and the milk a mother produces when her baby is two weeks old is different from the milk she creates when it is six months old.[1]

Formula lacks 100 of the identified components of human breast milk (and the list keeps growing as research continues).[2]

The immune system of breastfed babies is more efficient. Formula-fed babies had an 80 percent greater incidence of infections.

Breastfed babies have one-seventh as many allergies as formula-fed babies.[3]

BREASTFEEDING IS GOOD FOR MUMS TOO!

Mothers also benefit physically and emotionally from breastfeeding. Having your baby suckle at your breast contracts your womb, helps it and your entire body return to its prebirth state … It has now been shown that breastfeeding causes a woman's body to produce special hormones that calm her.[4]

DON'T WORRY! DON'T SUPPLEMENT WITH FORMULA!

Most baby growth charts are based on data from formula-fed babies. Between three and 12 months, breastfed babies grow more slowly than formula-fed infants.

INTRODUCING A BACK-UP BOTTLE

I generally do not encourage breastfeeding-on-demand to the *exclusion* of supplemental bottlefeeding. In these days of working mothers, breastfeeding-on-demand for many months can be unrealistic. The isolation and demands of parenting in a nuclear or single-parent family, and in a society which often forces mothers to return to work in the first months postpartum, can overwhelm the best intentions of a breastfeeding mother. Breastfeeding-on-demand can be done, but if it's causing guilt, stress, and undue hardship, a back-up bottle may be a solution. Breastfeeding should be a joy, not a burden.

Once a baby learns to take a bottle, I encourage fathers to bottle-feed their baby one time during the night (at least a few times a week) to let the mum get a desperately-needed four to five hours of uninterrupted sleep. This kind of support can help stave off postpartum depression, while nurturing the marital relationship.

So, in order to take better care of yourself during the stressful postpartum period, introduce the baby to a bottle between 3 and 4 weeks of age. A baby often refuses a bottle from its nursing mother, but will readily accept it from someone else. Some babies fuss if they can see, hear, or smell their mother in the room, so this is a good time for you to take that bath or nap you've been fantasizing about.

Bottlefeeding takes less effort and requires a different kind of sucking than does breastfeeding. So, bottlefeeding before three weeks may cause "nipple confusion," which means the baby develops a preference for sucking on the bottle and loses interest in breastfeeding. In the past, mothers were advised not to introduce the bottle until six weeks postpartum to avoid nipple confusion, but most babies will refuse the bottle by then! By three to four weeks, babies are used to breastfeeding (and prefer it) but remain open-minded about accepting an occasional alternative.

So, begin by offering an ounce or two (30–60ml) of breastmilk (or formula) in a bottle *once a day*. Since babies have short memories, do it *every* day for several weeks—or they will forget that a bottle is an acceptable alternative.

The best time to introduce a bottle is in the evening, when less breast milk is produced and your baby might like a little extra. Begin offering the bottle when your baby is awake, relaxed and between feedings. If your baby is starving and screaming (and isn't yet familiar with the bottle), try calming your baby by giving an "appetizer" (i.e., a brief breastfeeding). After your baby is calm, offer the bottle.

If you have frozen pumped breastmilk, thaw it in a bowl of warm tap water. Don't overheat it or microwave it—overheating destroys important elements in breastmilk. If you are using formula follow the directions on the container.

Warm the nipple under the tap so it's more like mother's nipple. Turn the bottle upside down to make sure it's not clogged—it should drip milk a drop a second.

Sit your baby upright (not lying on its back) to avoid flooding the baby. Try stroking the bottle nipple against the roof of the baby's mouth to elicit the sucking reflex.

If your baby won't take the bottle you're offering, try an *Avent* bottle. Many previously frustrated couples report immediate success after switching to an *Avent* bottle.

Even if you don't have to return to work during the first year, for a number of reasons you might be temporarily unavailable to nurse. Or you and your husband may want to go out on a date. A baby that knows how to take a bottle will be happier—and so will you!

BREAST ENGORGEMENT

Between the third and fifth day postpartum, some women experience swollen, hard, and painful breasts due to water retention and lymphatic engorgement (not an abundance of milk).

To relieve engorgement:

A. BEFORE NURSING:

Try warm baths, showers, or a heating pad to help your milk "let down." If your breasts are so full of milk the nipple is stretched flat, the baby won't be able to latch on. Before nursing, try expressing or pumping enough milk out to achieve an erect nipple.

B. IN BETWEEN NURSING:

Try cold cabbage leaves to reduce interstitial fluid/swelling (not your milk supply). Roll or crush the spines of cabbage leaves in your hands or under a rolling pin, then wear a cabbage leaf against each breast, tucked in your bra. Change every two hours. Frozen washcloths or ice packs placed against your breasts also bring relief.

— ANNIE FURIE, BSN, LACTATION CONSULTANT
OWNER OF *GROWING LIFE*, ALBUQUERQUE

Chapter 43

Preserving Your Birth Memories

The day you give birth you're sure this momentous event will be burned into your memory forever. And there *are* moments you will never forget. However, certain thoughts, images, and feelings begin to fade quickly after birth.

If you wish to preserve your birth memory, begin jotting down or sketching images within a few days after birth. You may be exhausted, anxious, and overwhelmed, but a few moments writing or drawing each day will be cherished later.

Include details about your birth such as the light in the room, the sound of rain on the roof, the moment you gathered up your greatest strength and determination, or the first time you saw your baby's face. Avoid writing a medical summary—write about *your* experience. Rebecca wrote her memory in a poem (page 362).

A journal can be kept at your bedside or carried easily in a nappy bag. When a ball point won't do to express a certain thought, image, or feeling, try coloured pens, pencils or magic markers.

Don't edit or try to create a literary masterpiece! Begin wherever you are and make entries whenever you want to preserve a memory (which may become a treasured heirloom).

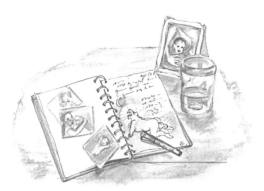

There are situations when even a brief entry may be too difficult. A friend told me she wasn't up to writing after her second baby was born with a birth defect requiring surgery. She used a tape recorder to capture her feelings during that trying experience, and saved the tape for him.

You may want to invite your partner, midwife, doctor, friends or the grandparents, to make entries in your journal. One mother included letters written by her own mother to her new baby.

Some memories can only be expressed in pictures. I had to sketch and paint what I felt just moments before and during Luc's birth.

If you regret not "recording" a previous birth, begin now by writing whatever memory comes to mind. One memory will lead you to another. Keep writing.

> Your hand against my foot lets me push past my fear through that small hole inside of myself my strength growing like crystals on glass exponentially, beautifully.
>
> Your warmth runs up my leg cocooning my belly calling to that small moth, that butterfly inside of me to emerge slowly uncurling her moist wings, hungry mouth into your cradlehand.
>
> You kneel waiting patiently for the rest to slide with an explosion of joy & wetness into your arms, my arms & together we laugh.
>
> – REBECCA MAYKETA

PHOTOGRAPHS AND VIDEO-TAPES

Weddings, graduations, and vacations are events typically celebrated with family, friends, and Kodak. Although having a baby is the ultimate family experience, it is also a private matter, which summons a willingness to be open, sexual, primal, even vulnerable. Photographing or video-taping of your birth should be done in a discreet and respectful manner.

The way a birth is video-taped is important. If you anticipate being stationary, a tripod can be set up in the corner of the room, where it becomes part of the background. This eliminates the need to have an extra person at your birth. I've seen several couples do this successfully.

Alternatively, you can ask a close and sensitive friend, who understands her position is to be unseen and unheard, to take your photos or video. Ideally she will have a flair for creative shots, without intruding on your awareness or asking you to "pose." As you drift into Labourland, you will be less aware of the camera. I've been at many births where the photographer's sensitivity resulted in a mother expressing regret that no pictures were taken. When told pictures *were* taken, she'd exclaim, "I never even heard the camera click! Who took the pictures?"

HOSPITAL/DOCTOR POLICY: NO PHOTOGRAPHS OR VIDEO-TAPING

Be aware that some doctors and hospitals strictly forbid "patients" taking photographs or videos during labour or birth for fear it might be used against them in litigation. Other doctors encourage photos during Caesarean birth! If you have your heart set on having birth photos/video, find out whether such restrictions exist, and if it's possible to obtain special permission—*before* you are in labour.

WARNING: SEEING OR LISTENING TO YOURSELF GIVE BIRTH MIGHT BE TRAUMATIC

> I couldn't wait to see the photos of my first labour. I opened the envelope as quickly as I could only to be shocked at the feeling that came over me when I saw them! Did I look like that?! Without warning, I instantly and *vividly* remembered what I had already started to forget—the pain, fear and disappointment. I quickly put away the photos and could not look at them for several years.
>
> HEATHER

Not everyone's experience is like Heather's. Some people love their birth photos and show them to everyone. But you can't predict what your reaction will be. The tips below may be worth considering before you open the envelope of photos.

A birth video can spotlight forgotten or unnoticed aspects of your birth, as well as intensify your sensory-memory of the experience. For some women, this can be a highly positive process, but for others it may be extremely traumatic. Watching, particularly listening to, a video recording of yourself giving birth can bring to conscious awareness memories nature intended to be forgotten.

Sujata had her first baby at home in her hot tub. It was a normal birth, lovingly supported in every way. The next day, before she had had time to make her own memory (this takes about three weeks), she watched her birth video.

> I don't think the trauma from that video healed until I had my second baby. Watching the video made me relive the pain again and again. I felt violated … watching the video made me angry, I felt betrayed by God … It was so painful.

When asked what was the hardest part of watching the video of Antonio's birth, Sujata quickly said, "The sound was the hardest part. I watched it several times … it was a lot easier to watch with the sound off."

With video, your memory of your birth becomes an out-of-body image as you *observe* yourself giving birth—instead of remembering it from within, from being *in* birth. A video can also reduce an experience by superimposing the dimension of linear time onto an experience where it didn't exist (when you were floating in Labourland).

*

A few years later, Sujata had another baby at home. Here's how she compared her memories of her two births:

> Chelsea's birth was painful but the pain disappeared into the fog, so I only remember the bliss. When I think of Chelsea's birth, I think of the candles, and the warm water … but with Antonio I still remember the sounds I made when I pushed him out. I relive what I saw and heard on the tape.

Interestingly, they taped Chelsea's birth and "put it under lock and key." Sujata says she won't ever watch it, or let anyone else watch it, but is saving it for Chelsea in case she wants to watch it when she's grown up. "It'll be up to Chelsea to decide when and if to watch her birth tape."

- Wait at least six months, even a year, before viewing your birth video. Let your memory of birth be formed naturally.
- Anticipate the possibility of a vast range of emotions while watching your video: embarrassment, love, pride, joy, shame, sadness or fear.
- Be with someone who loves you, whom you can talk to if the video does upset you.
- Be selective about whom you share your video with. Many women have shared their regrets about not anticipating the unprotected feeling of exposure they experienced after showing it to lots of people. Sujata sent a copy of her video for someone to edit, who casually showed it to some acquaintances. A year later, those people met Sujata and greeted her with, "Oh it's you, we saw the birth of your son …" Sujata felt violated, "I didn't even know these people, and they had seen me in my most vulnerable, private moments."
- Sometimes it's helpful to have your midwife watch with you to explain parts of the birth you don't understand.
- Turn down the sound. Just watch the birth.

Afterword

BIRTH AS AN ADVENTURE

One perfect October weekend Rob and I were in Georgia O'Keeffe country in northern New Mexico. We decided to go exploring. We had gotten a recommendation from the friendly folks at the Abiquiu Inn to try a hiking trail near the Muslim mosque overlooking the Chama River.

Below us, the river's course was traced by a golden blaze of cottonwoods lining its banks. We wandered off a rocky, dirt road towards what appeared to be a canyon, marked by chalky-white, otherworldly cliffs. We ventured ahead, uncertain about what we would encounter. The canyon narrowed, seemingly with every few steps, and our walk became a climb.

The moist earth changed to a sparkling trickle, then a small stream, as we followed it upward. The ascent became even steeper as the canyon narrowed further. Our progress now depended on precise placement of our feet and pushing off each white canyon wall with our arms.

Thunder began rumbling ominously. Looking up through the narrow slit above, we could see dark clouds gathering. Propelled by the image of our serene hiking trail becoming a raging sluice-way, we began scrambling back down. Big drops were falling and our hearts were racing as we reached the open valley below.

We were exhilarated by the thrill of having ventured into unknown terrain and faced a challenge, and pleased by having created a memory together.

Just as there are many ways to explore unknown territory, there are countless paths for you to take through pregnancy and birth. The most rewarding outcomes tend to spring from an openness to the unpredictable, and a mindset that embraces it all.

DRAWING ON WHAT YOU HAVE LEARNED

I often ask couples taking my Birthing From Within classes to talk about the most significant thing they learned during the classes, and how it will help them. Sometimes I ask them to make a drawing of that to have with them during labour.

So, when you've finished working with this book, take a few moments to reflect on what was most useful or inspirational, and express it in writing or art. People have told me how important reminders like these can be when things get tough in labour.

*

> "Thus we cover the universe
> with drawings we have lived."
>
> – GASTON BACHELARD

We'd love to hear about your birth experiences, and reactions to our book. Your feedback will help us make an even better second edition for future parents.

No matter how your birth unfolds, or what surprises it brings, we wish you a great Birth From Within.

Pam England
Rob Horowitz
c/o Partera Press
P.O. Box 4528
Albuquerque, NM 87106

Appendix A

SPECIAL DIETS FOR SPECIAL CONDITIONS

"WHAT SHOULD I DO IF I'M CARRYING TWINS?"

You need 120–140 grams of protein and 3,100 calories every day to carry healthy twins to term. Often twin babies are born early and/or small because the mother was not eating enough.

*

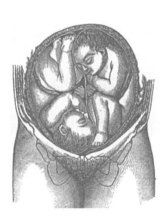

"I DON'T LIKE MILK" OR "I'M ALLERGIC TO MILK."

During pregnancy and breastfeeding you need 1,200 mg calcium, or the equivalent of one litre of milk, every day. Your baby soaks up 85 percent of the calcium you take into your body to form healthy teeth and bones. Over half of the calcium present in your baby's body at birth is absorbed during the last two months of pregnancy.

Beyond its important calcium contribution, milk provides essential protein. If you do not consume any dairy products, you will need to make up about 30 grams of protein, in *addition* to your two servings of meat, beans, tofu, etc.

Calcium-Rich Foods: Calcium is present in cheese, sardines, seaweed, leafy greens, sesame seeds and molasses.

If you simply don't like the taste of milk, try a milk shake with ice cream, fruit, or protein powder.

Supplements: You can also ensure you're getting enough calcium by taking calcium-magnesium supplements.

Warning: If you are a lacto-ovo vegetarian: you will need to take a B-12 supplement, because vitamin B-12 is found almost exclusively in dairy/animal products. Besides causing anaemia, vitamin B-12 deficiency is associated with brain and neurological damage in newborns. One vegetarian food source of this vitamin is tempeh, a fermented soy product.

*

PUMPING IRON

Extra iron is necessary for foetal blood development and to build a three to four month reserve of iron in the baby's liver. This iron bank protects a breastfed baby from anaemia, until the baby is able to get iron from solid food.

Extra iron is also needed to build up maternal iron reserves in order to protect the mother from the effects of blood loss at birth.

FOLIC ACID

In the United States approximately 2,500 babies are born each year with neural tube defects, including spina bifida. By taking 0.4 to 1.0 mg of folic acid daily in the beginning of pregnancy (or even before), you can expect to reduce that risk by 50 to 70 percent.

During pregnancy you need 18 to 20 mg of iron daily to make good, strong blood for both you and your baby. Did you know that during the second half of pregnancy your blood volume *doubles*? This ensures healthy circulation of oxygen and nutrients to your baby through the placenta, and protects against shock from normal blood loss during delivery. During the last four months of pregnancy, your baby needs up to 7.5 mg iron every day (to build up its iron stores for the first six months of life).

With attention to your diet and proper supplements, you can expect to see a significant rise in your haemoglobin (blood iron levels) within two to three weeks.

IRON *SUPPLEMENTS*:

Non-pregnant women need 18 mg of iron daily. But, during pregnancy, you and your baby need 30–60 mg of supplemental iron daily. Even if your diet is iron-rich, it may not be adequate, since only 10 to 20 percent of ingested iron is absorbed into the bloodstream.

Medieval physicians treated anaemia by having the patient drink blood. Fortunately, you don't need to depend on that Transylvanian treatment. Extra iron may be prescribed by your doctor or midwife (to be taken in addition to your prenatal vitamin). Usually, 75–100 mg chelated iron once or twice a day (depending on the degree of anaemia) will resolve anaemia in a month. You might prefer a food-source liquid iron/herbal supplement called Floridex.

Generally speaking, mineral supplements are difficult to absorb, and iron supplements often cause constipation. To avoid this problem, try *chelated* iron. Chelation is a process whereby minerals are bound with an amino acid, which the body readily recognizes. The right enzyme to break down and absorb the minerals is then produced. Therefore, chelated iron is absorbed through the intestines three times more readily than ordinary ferous sulfate. Chelated minerals are available at herb and health food stores.

IRON-RICH FOODS INCLUDE: liver, organ and red meats (try to buy organic organ meats), seaweed, soybeans, red kidney beans, molasses, prune juice, raisins, dried apricots and most dried fruits (except dried apples).

VITAMIN C (250 mg) taken with iron supplements *doubles the absorption of iron* by increasing hydrochloric acid in the stomach (during pregnancy hydrochloric acid in the stomach is decreased). Orange juice is not a good substitute for a vitamin C supplement because its sugar neutralizes the acid in the stomach.

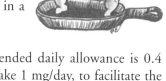

Cooking in an iron skillet significantly increases the iron content of food, especially acidic foods such as tomatoes. Acidic food seems to coax iron out of a skillet. For example, a tomato that has 3 mg of iron is "pumped up" to 87 mg after stewing in a cast-iron pot for a few hours.

FOLIC ACID: The minimum recommended daily allowance is 0.4 mg/day. However, you may want to take 1 mg/day, to facilitate the development of red blood cells.

FOLIC ACID FOOD SOURCES INCLUDE:

Green leafy vegies such as spinach (the darker the better), dried beans, peas, lentils, citrus fruits, and whole grain bread and cereals.

WHAT IS GESTATIONAL DIABETES? HOW CAN A SPECIAL DIET HELP?

During pregnancy the body undergoes various changes in carbohydrate metabolism. Insulin, a hormone produced by the pancreas, regulates the amount of sugar in the blood. Specific pregnancy hormones, however, block the action of insulin. When this happens, women usually produce more insulin to maintain a stable blood sugar level. Unfortunately, women predisposed to diabetes can't produce that extra insulin. Sugar in their urine or a high blood sugar level are clues that they have developed gestational diabetes.

About five percent of women develop diabetes during pregnancy. Usually it is mild, managed by diet, and clears up after delivery.

Another indication of possible gestational diabetes is a baby which is growing unusually rapidly. When a mother's blood sugar is too high, her baby gets the overflow. Sugar in the mother's blood quickly crosses the placental barrier and enters the baby's bloodstream. The baby produces its own insulin, so the higher its blood sugar, the more insulin the baby produces. Increased insulin allows greater amounts of sugar to be absorbed into the baby's cells, where it is used either for energy or stored as fat. Because a baby's energy needs are limited, the extra sugar results in a fat baby. Sometimes babies born to mothers with gestational diabetes weigh 9,10, even 12 or more pounds at birth. Of course, not all babies over eight pounds are born of diabetic mothers—some women just have big babies!

If the mother's blood sugar level is not controlled, here's what may happen to the baby after birth: Immediately after the baby is born and the umbilical cord is cut, its flow of sugar stops. Because the baby is still producing insulin, the baby's blood sugar level plummets. If left untreated, hypoglycemia (low blood sugar) could cause permanent brain damage.

A blood test is available to determine whether or not you have gestational diabetes. If you do, your doctor or midwife will refer you to a dietician. Follow the British Diabetic Association diet prescribed for you. By following that special diet, your blood sugar level likely will remain stable, and within normal limits.

WHAT IF MY BABY IS SMALLER THAN IT SHOULD BE AT THIS POINT IN PREGNANCY?

Check your diet against the *Common Sense Diet* outlined on page 34. You will probably discover that you and your baby have been needing more protein and calories. Follow that diet, and if you are smoking, cut back, or quit. Unless there is another underlying problem, your baby will begin to grow again.

*

Pre-eclampsia is a condition characterized by high blood pressure, abnormal swelling, and protein in the urine. It develops during the latter half of pregnancy, often in women whose diet is low in protein, calories, and salt. Inadequate nutrition restricts the normal growth of the placenta, baby, and mother's blood volume, which is then manifested as symptoms of pre-eclampsia.

A pregnant woman's blood volume doubles by the 28th week of pregnancy. Maintaining this tremendous volume is possible due to increased activity of the body's salt and water retention mechanisms. Also essential is a high-protein diet that allows her to make extra albumin.

Albumin is an important protein synthesized in the liver (provided the mother is eating an adequate amount of protein). Albumin retains proper amounts of fluid in the bloodstream. If albumin decreases, fluid that should be in the blood vessels is drawn from the blood into the surrounding tissues and causes swelling (edema).

Reduced blood volume results in a decreased flow to the kidneys, placenta and baby. The kidneys detect the low blood volume and sound an alarm, releasing a hormone, renin, into the bloodstream. Renin triggers the release of other hormones which, in turn, cause small arteries throughout the body to constrict. During a healthy pregnancy, progesterone actually relaxes blood vessels to allow for the increased volume of blood. But in pre-eclampsia, the body attempts to reduce the blood vessel capacity to match the lower volume. The result is high blood pressure.

PREVENTION IS BEST

A sound diet prevents pre-eclampsia. If you have mild symptoms, or a high haematocrit, begin improving your diet right away, and you may be able turn back the tide. Once pre-eclampsia has a foothold, there's no turning it back. You may wind up needing hospitalization and aggressive treatment.

First, check your daily intake against the COMMON SENSE DIET. You will probably discover you are lacking in protein and calories. During the first few weeks, eat 80–100 gms of protein a day. Once your symptoms resolve, maintain a well-balanced diet of 70–80 gms a day and 2,600 calories.

Appendix B

Before 32 weeks, at any given time 50 percent of babies are in breech position. However, as pregnancy progresses the baby's head becomes heavier than its bottom, and at around 32 weeks it usually sinks into the pelvis.

If between 32–35 weeks, your BA tells you your baby is breech, try turning your baby with the Breech Tilt exercise (which is usually more than 80 percent effective). Here's how to do it:

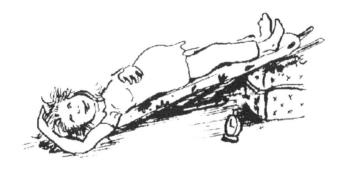

Lie on the floor and use cushions to elevate your hips to about a 30 degree angle, or lie on an ironing board propped up on the couch. It seems that the inverted postion helps the baby's bottom fall away from the pelvic brim, so when you stand up the "floating" baby can turn—led by the heavy head sinking downward.

Tilt for 10–15 minutes, two to three times a day, until the baby flips.

Simultaneously, try playing music or buzzing your electric tooth brush against the abdomen. In one study 15 out of 16 foetuses in the breech positon turned around upon hearing the buzzing of an artificial larynx device.

If your baby is still breech at 36–37 weeks, your doctor may suggest *external version* to manually turn the baby (70–90 percent success rate).

Your breech tilt can be even more effective if you practise deep abdominal-pelvic relaxation through visualization or hypnosis. Lewis Mehl (1994) taught 100 mothers with breech-babies relaxation through self-hypnosis. At delivery 81 of the babies had turned head-down; in contrast only 48 babies of the 100 women in the control group (who hadn't learned relaxation through visualization) had turned![1]

Appendix C

WORKSHEETS FOR LEARNING PAIN-COPING TECHNIQUES

These worksheets may be reproduced by parents for their personal use. Written permission is required for commercial reproduction, publication, or education.

BASELINE OF PAIN (PAGE 284)

Rate the sensation of pain when holding the ice:

0____1____2____3____4____5____6____7____8____9____10
      BARELY   NOTICEABLE   INTENSE
  NOTICEABLE   BUT MANAGEABLE   INTOLERABLE

Notes:

BREATH AWARENESS (PAGE 285)

WHILE PRACTISING BREATH AWARENESS, RATE THE INTENSITY OF ICE-PAIN:

0____1____2____3____4____5____6____7____8____9____10
      BARELY   NOTICEABLE   INTENSE
  NOTICEABLE   BUT MANAGEABLE   INTOLERABLE

Using the 1–10 scale above, rate the sensation of pain when you practise the following variations:

WHAT HAPPENS WHEN YOU LET GO OF YOUR IDEAS OR MEMORY OF PAIN AND JUST NOTICE HOW THE INTENSITY AND LOCATION OE THE SENSATION CHANGE WITH EACH BREATH OUT?

HOW DOES ADDING IMAGINATION (VISUALIZATION) CHANGE THE INTENSITY OF PAIN? (PAGE 286)

NON-FOCUSED AWARENESS (NFA—PAGES 287–294)

Score the effectiveness of NFA by rating the intensity of ice-pain:

0____1____2____3____4____5____6____7____8____9____10
  BARELY   NOTICEABLE   INTENSE
NOTICEABLE   BUT MANAGEABLE   INTOLERABLE

Notes:

Using the 1–10 scale above, rate the effectiveness of NFA while practising the following variations:

VERBAL/NON-VERBAL SHIFTING (PAGE 290)

1) Saying silently to yourself what you are noticing

2) Saying aloud what you are noticing

3) While being cued through NFA by your birth partner:
   a) Notice silently what you are noticing
   b) Say aloud what you are noticing.

QUAKER LISTENING (PAGE 290)

Give your birth partner feedback and suggestions on how he/she guided you. Were the suggestions too specific (e.g., you were told *what* to notice)? Was the pace about right? Make a note about what works best. Try it again after reviewing tips on cuing on pages 291.

What happens when you add music or nature sounds?

EYES OPEN OR CLOSED?

Using NFA or Quaker Listening, see if there is a difference when your eyes are open or closed?

VARY YOUR PACE (OF NOTICING)

Does speeding up or slowing down work better for you at different levels of pain intensity?

INTRODUCE DISTRACTION

Rate how well you were able to maintain concentration on NFA while your birth partner or childbirth teacher purposefully creates a distraction (e.g., noise, talking loudly, touching you).

0____1____2____3____4____5____6____7____8____9____10
     BARELY   NOTICEABLE   INTENSE
   NOTICEABLE   BUT MANAGEABLE   INTOLERABLE

Did the distraction deepen or disturb your concentration? Why?

Imagine being distracted in labour. Talk about what you and your birth partner will need to do to stay on track. Make a note of these ideas to remind you when you're in labour.

EDGES (PAGES 294–296)

Rate the effectiveness of practising Edges of Pain:

0____1____2____3____4____5____6____7____8____9____10
    BARELY   NOTICEABLE   INTENSE
  NOTICEABLE   BUT MANAGEABLE   INTOLERABLE

Notes:

USING THE 1 – 10 SCALE ABOVE, RATE THE EFFECTIVENESS WHILE PRACTISING THE FOLLOWING VARIATIONS OF EDGES:

EDGES OF COMFORT (PAGE 295)

Do a body scan focusing on what parts of your body are *not* in pain.

PAIN UNDER A MAGNIFYING GLASS (PAGE 296)

SOFTENING AROUND THE EDGES

Give your birth partner feedback on the guided imagery (page 224). Which metaphor or images worked? Do you have suggestions for images or phrases that might be helpful? Was the pace too fast, too slow, or just right? Try again. Write the images or phrases that worked best below.

FINDING THE CENTRE (PAGES 297–298)

Rate the effectiveness of Centre by rating the intensity of ice-pain:

0____1____2____3____4____5____6____7____8____9____10
    BARELY   NOTICEABLE   INTENSE
  NOTICEABLE   BUT MANAGEABLE   INTOLERABLE

Notes:

TRICKLING OUT THE PAIN

As you breathe out, imagine the sensation and all your ideas about it slowly trickling out through a tiny opening in the centre of the sensation, like grains of sand floating out into the infinite universe.

BREATHING INTO THE CENTRE

What happens when you breathe right into the centre of the sensation with deliberate, slow, and forceful exhalations?

See what happens when you breathe faster.

   Breathe the centre *in* on your inhalation; and/or *move* the centre with your exhalation, like an armadillo pushing a beach ball with its snout.

SPIRALLING (PAGE 298)

Rate the intensity of ice-pain while practising Spiralling:

0____1____2____3____4____5____6____7____8____9____10
   BARELY   NOTICEABLE   INTENSE
NOTICEABLE   BUT MANAGEABLE   INTOLERABLE

Notes:

SPIRALLING USING THE FOLLOWING VARIATIONS:

CHANCE THE DIRECTION AND/OR PLANE OF THE SPIRAL.

STOP THE SPIRAL'S MOVEMENT AS YOU BREATHE IN, AND MOVE THE SPIRAL AS YOU BREATHE OUT.

WHAT HAPPENS WHEN YOU CHANGE THE SPEED OF THE SPIRALLING?

FINDING YOUR VOICE (PAGES 300–304)

Hold a piece of ice and begin rhythmically to chant a phrase or make a sound. Try to merge your voice with the sensation of ice; moan the sound or words from deep in your belly.

HOW DID EXPRESSING SOUND INFLUENCE THE SENSATION OF THE ICE?

WHAT OTHER CHANGES IN YOUR EMOTIONS OR PHYSICAL SENSATIONS DID YOU NOTICE?

CO-CHANTING (PAGE 304)

FATHER OR BIRTH COMPANION:

Listen to her vocal-pattern, then chant with her.

TRY COMBINING CO-CHANTING WITH TOUCH-RELAXATION (PAGES 304–306). SHARE FEEDBACK AND SUGGESTIONS.

WHAT EFFECT DID CO-CHANTING HAVE ON YOUR SELFCONSCIOUSNESS ABOUT MAKING, OR HEARING, BIRTHING SOUNDS? AS A MOTHER DID YOU FEEL MORE SUPPORTED OR ACCEPTED? AS A FATHER, DID YOU FEEL MORE SUPPORTIVE AND ACCEPTING?

IF CO-CHANTING WAS A DISTRACTION (TO THE MOTHER), IS THERE ANYTHING YOUR PARTNER COULD DO DIFFERENTLY? TRY IT.

IN WHAT WAYS HAS YOUR ATTITUDE ABOUT WOMEN BEING VOCAL IN LABOUR CHANGED AS A RESULT OF THIS EXERCLSE?

Appendix D

These pocket-reminder cards are intended for private use by parents. Permission to reproduce these cards for publication or education must be obtained in writing from authors.

HELPFUL REMINDERS FOR FATHERS AND OTHER BIRTH COMPANIONS

REMEMBER THE IMPORTANCE OF:

- Protect privacy, turn off phone, close door, restrict visitors. Birth is not a happening/She is not a party hostess.
- Observe/anticipate her needs. Don't ask too many questions.
- Respectful silence, or talk to her slowly, softly during contractions.
- Use non-verbal signals.
- Suggest bath or shower, change in position, walking, voiding.
- Encourage sips of nutritive drink, at least a quarter of a pint per hour. Choose sports drinks, tea with honey, juice (not just water/ice chips).
- Wear the hide of an encyclopaedia salesman—don't take any rejection or reaction personally.

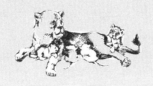

PAIN-COPING TECHNIQUES

REMEMBER:

- Be curious about the pain
- Notice what's already working ... and do more of that
- Breath Awareness
- Build a Partnership With Your Baby
- Non-Focused Awareness (mindful awareness without judging)
- Quaker Listening
- Edges of Sensation
- Edges of Comfort (Where exactly does the sensation begin and end? How does it move/change with each breath out?)
- Centre of Sensation (emptiness/stillness in the eye of the hurricane)
- Spiralling (out of the centre of sensation, moving the spiral with each exhalation)
- Touch Awareness (downward stroke on her outward breath)
- Massage
- Primordial Vocalization or Co-chanting

QUESTIONS TO HELP YOU GET INFORMATION*

TESTS AND PROCEDURES:

- What will we find out from this test/procedure?
- How accurate is it?
- What are the risks?
- Do they outweigh the benefits?
- What will you or we do differently based on the results?
- If nothing, is there another reason to do it?

TREATMENTS, DRUGS AND INTERVENTIONS:

- How will this be helpful?
- Why must this be done now? What might happen if we wait an hour? A week? Or do nothing?
- What are the advantages/disadvantages?
- This may be the treatment you usually recommend, but what other approaches can you tell us about?
- If several treatment choices are possible: Is there a logical sequence in which to try the different options?

Appendix E

Circumcision
(continued from pages 250–251.)

(continued from pages 250–251.)

WHY DID CIRCUMCISION BECOME SO COMMON IN AMERICA?

"During the 20th century in the United States, the majority of males have been circumcised as newborns, usually before leaving the hospital after birth. The practice originated as a result of the anti-masturbation hysteria of the late 1800's. People feared that if a boy had a foreskin and had to pull it back while cleaning his penis he would learn to masturbate. At that time it was believed that masturbation led to insanity."[1]

Another reason circumcision was widely promoted in the 19th century was the now-discredited belief that it would protect men from sexually transmitted diseases.

SO WHY ARE BABIES STILL BEING CIRCUMCISED?

Although the rate of newborn circumcision has been steadily declining over the past two decades, 40–60 percent of baby boys still undergo this painful surgical procedure, often with no anaesthesia. Underlying this practice is the implicit assumption that nature has somehow "goofed" in its design for little boys.

Research has dispelled the myths which still perpetuate the tradition of newborn circumcision: it's needed to maintain genital hygiene; it significantly decreases risk of infections or penile cancer; it's a painless procedure for babies; and it prevents trauma from not "Looking-Like-Daddy" or the other kids in the locker room.

Of course, religious customs have also been part of parents choosing newborn circumcision. Parents need to decide whether those customs are sufficient justification in the absence of other compelling reasons for this procedure.

WHAT IF YOU ARE STILL UNDECIDED?

Arrange to see another baby undergo circumcision. Many parents who are ambivalent, but decide to allow the procedure, later regret it. They've told me they wished they had known what their baby (and they) were going to have to endure.

IF YOU DO DECIDE TO HAVE YOUR BABY CIRCUMCISED ...

Stay with him during the procedure, talk to him. Try to nurse and cuddle him afterward.

FOR MORE INFORMATION ON CIRCUMCISION AND FORESKIN HYGIENE, WRITE:

NORM-UK, PO Box 71, Stone, Staffordshire, ST15 0SF (tel: 0175 814044; www.norm-uk.org)

www.nhsdirect.nhs.uk (tel: 0845 4647)

NOTES

CHAPTER 2: EMPTYING THE MIND

1 Epigraph on page 6: Baker, Richard (1970). Introduction to *Zen mind, beginner's mind* by Shunryo Suzuki. New York and Tokyo: Weatherhill.
2 *Ibid*, pp. 13–14. (Poem on page 8)

CHAPTER 3: WORRY IS THE WORK OF PREGNANCY

Epigraph on page 11: Rabuzzi, Kathryn Allen (1988). *Motherself: A mythic analysis of motherhood* p. 204. Bloomington, Indiana: Indiana University Press.

CHAPTER 4: CONNECTING WITH WOMEN

Epigraph on page 19: Kent, Corita and Stewart, Jan (1992). *Learning by heart: Teachings to free the creative spirit* p. 198. New York: Bantam Books.
1 Panuthos, Claudia (1984). *Transformation through birth.* p. 132. Massachusetts: Begin and Garvey.
2 Dunham, Carroll and the Body Shop Team (1991). *Mamatoto: A celebration of birth* p. 58. New York: Viking.
3 Kent, C. and Stewart, J. *op. cit.* p. 200.
4 Sale, Robin (1992). Creating a blessing way ceremony. *The Doula.* Winter. pp. 12–14.
5 Cooper, Patricia and Buferd, Norma Bradley (1978). *The quilters: women and domestic art* pp. 22–24. Garden City, New York: Anchor Press/Doubleday.
   Epigraph on page 23: Wigginton, Eliot, Editor (1968) *The Foxfire Book.* p. 149. A quilt is something human. Garden City, New York: Anchor/Doubleday.
6 *Ibid*, p. 148.

CHAPTER 5: EATING IN AWARENESS

1 David Stewart (1981). *The five standards for safe childbearing* pp. 105–106. Marble Hill, Missouri: NAPSAC Reproductions.
2 Audio tape of Thich Nhat Hanh (1990). *Peace making: How to be it, how to do it.* Boulder, Colorado: Sounds True Recordings.
3 Thich Nhat Hanh (1988). *The heart of understanding* pp. 3–4. Berkeley, California: Parallax Press.

CHAPTER 8: TAKING THE PLUNGE

1 Da Vinci, Leonardo, quoted in Jung, Carl (1984). *Man and his symbols.* New York: Dell Publishers, p. 10.
2 Naumberg Cane, Florence (1951). *The artist in each of us.* New York: Pantheon.

CHAPTER 9: DISCOVERY THROUGH DRAWING

Epigraph on page 54: Harding, Esther M. (1939). *The way of all women.* New York: I.ongmans, Green and Co.
1 Chicago, Judy (1979). *The Birth Project* p. 73. Garden City, New York: Doubleday Anchor Press.
2 French, Marilyn (1977). *The Women's Room* pp. 49–50. New York: Summit Books.

CHAPTER 11: REVELATIONS THROUGH CLAY

1 Sjoo, Monica and Mor, Barbara (1987). *The Great Cosmic Mother* p. 84. New York: Harper and Row.
2 Neumann, Erich (1963). *The Great Mother: An analysls of the archetype* p. 96. New York: Bolligen Foundation.
3 Sjoo, Monica and Mor, Barbara *op. cit* p. 17.
Epigraph on page 81: Berensohn, Paulus (1972). *Finding one's way with clay* p. 146. New York: Simon and Schuster.
Epigraph on page 87: Griffin, Susan (1978). *Woman and nature* p. 227. New York: Harper Colophon Books.

CHAPTER 13: BIRTH ART INSIGHTS FROM PROFESSIONAL ARTISTS

1 Craighead, Meinrad (1986). *The mother songs: Images of god the mother* p. 66. New York: Paulist Press.
2 *Ibid*, p. i.
3 Chicago, Judy (1979). *The birth project* p. 6. Garden City, New York: Doubleday Anchor Press.
4 Gadon, Elinor (1989). *The once and future goddess: A symbol of our time* p. 8. New York: Harper and Row.

CHAPTER 15: WHERE MOTHERS BUILD THEIR NESTS

1 Rich, Adrienne quoted in Eakins, Pamela S.(1986). *The American way of birth* p. 3. Philadelphia: Temple University Press.
2 Weigle, Marta (1989). Creation and procreation: Feminist reflections on mythologies on cosmogeny and parturition. University of Pennsylvania Press, p. 206.
3 Sorel, Nancy Caldwell (1984). *Ever since Eve* pp. 114–115. New York: Oxford University Press.
4 Graham, Judy (1977). A place to breath. *Nursing Times.* November 20:28–29.

5 Starkman M.N. (1976). Psychological responses to the use of the foetal monitor during labor. *Psychosomatic Medicine* 38, July/Aug:269–78.

CHAPTER 16: CHILDBIRTH AS A RITE OF PASSAGE

1 Bates, Brian and Turner, Allison Newman (1985). Imagery and symbolism in the birth practices of traditional cultures. *Birth* vol. 12 (1), Spring:31.
2 *Ibid*, p.32.
3 *Ibid*, p.32.

CHAPTER 19: HOME BIRTH

1 Hannon, Sharron (1990). *Childbirth: A source book* p. 150. New York: M. Evans and Company, Inc.
2 Goer, Henci (1995). *Obstetric myths versus research realities: A guide to the medical literature* pp. 335–336. Westport, Connecticut: Bergin & Garvey.
3 Reading, Anthony (1983). *Psychological aspects of pregnancy* p. 8. New York: Longman.
4 Goer, Henci. *op. cit* p. 334.
5 Campbell, Rona (1990). The place of birth. In *Intrapartum care: A research-based approach* pp. 1–23. Great Britain: The Macmillan Press LTD.
6 Goer, Henci. *op. cit* p. 332.
7 Devitt, Neal (1977). The transition from home to hospital birth in the United States, 1930–1960. *Birth and the Family Journal*, vol. 4:2, Summer 1977:47–57.
8 Tew, Marjorie (1985). Ilome births. *Nursing Times*, November 20: 24.
9 Hannon, Sharron (1980). *Childbirth: A source book for conception, pregnancy, birth and the first weeks of life* p. 52. New York: M. Evans and Company, Inc. '
10 Duran, AM. (1992). The safety of home birth: The Farm study. *American Iournal of Public Health*, vol 82 (3):450–453.
11 Mehl, Lewis, Peterson, Gayle, Witt, Michael, and Hawes, Warren E. (1977). Outcomes of elective home births: a series of 1,146 cases. *Journal of Reproductive Medicine*. vol. 19,(5):281–290.
12 Mehl, Lewis (1976). From a lecture presented to The American Foundation for Maternal and Infant Health.
13 Sullivan, Deborah and Beeman, Ruth (1983). Four years experience with home birth by licensed midwives in Arizona. *American Journal of Public Health*. vol. 73, No. 6, June:641–645.
14 Fleissig, Anne and Cartwright, Ann (1992). Women's preference for place of birth. *British Medical Journal*, vol 305, Aug 22, letters to editor.
15 Albers, Leah (1994). Electronic fetal monitoring reassessed. *Childbirth Instructor Magazine*. Winter:24–27.
16 Goer, Henci (1995). *op. cit* p. 334.

CHAPTER 21: LABOUR MEANS HARD WORK

1 Armstrong, Penny and Feldman, Sheryl (1986). *A midwifes story* pp. 5962. New York: Arbor House.

2 Lee, Martin, Lee, Emily, Lee, Melinda, Lee, Joyce (© 1996). *The healing art of tai chi: Becoming one with nature* pp. 22–23. Reprinted with permission of Sterling Publishing Co., Inc., 387 Park Ave. S., N.Y., N.Y. 10016.

3 Diamond, Susan L. (1996). *Hard Labor* p. 58. New York: Forge.

CHAPTER 22: OUT OF CONTROL: HOW TO "LOSE IT" IN LABOR

1 Gangaji (1995). Audiotape of Satsang: "The Freedom of No Escape." July 6 in Boulder, Colorado. Satsang Foundation & Press, Boulder, Colorado.

CHAPTER 23: THESE BONES WERE MADE FOR BIRTHIN'

Gaskin, Ina May (1978) *Spiritual midwifery.* Summertown, Tennessee: The Book Publishing Company.

1 Limburg, Astrid and Smulders, Beatrijs (1992). *Women giving birth* pp. 56. Berkeley, California: Celestial Arts.

2 Ollendorf, David et al (1988). Vaginal birth after cesarean section for arrest of labor: Is success determined by maximum cervical dilation during the prior labor? *American Journal Obstetrics and Gynecology*, 159:636–639.

3 Prickhardt, Mark et al (1992). Vaginal birth after cesarean delivery: Are there useful and valid predictors of success or failure? *Obstetrics and Gynecology*, 166:1811–1819.

4 Rosen, Mortimer and Dickinson, Janet C. (1990). Vaginal birth after cesarean: A meta-analysis of indicators for success. *Obstetrics and Gynecology*, 76:865–869.

CHAPTER 24: STAND AND DELIVER

1 Hamilton. G. (1861). Classical observations and suggestions in obstetrics. *Edinburgh Medical lournal.* 7:313–321 quoted in Barnett and Humenick (1982). Infant outcome in relation to second stage labor pushing method. *Birth*, 9:4,Winter:221.

2 Caldeyro-Barcia, Roberto (1979). The influence of maternal bearing down efforts during second stage on fetal well-being. *Birth and the Family lournal*, vol. 6:1, Spring:17–21.

3 Barnett, Mary M. and Humenick, Sharron (1982). Infant outcome in relation to second stage labor pushing method. *Birth* vol. 9:4, Winter:221–225.

4 Caldeyro-Barcia, Roberto (1979). *op. cit.* pp. 7–15.

5 Chou Liu, Yuen (1979). Position during labor and delivery: history and perspective. *Journal of Nurse-Midwifery*, vol. 24, No.3, May/June:23–26.

6 Caldeyro-Barcia, Roberto (1979). *op. cit* p. 7.

7 Limberg, Astrid and Smulders, Beatrijs (1990). *op. cit.* p. 4.

8 Pritchard and McDonald (1993).19th ed. *Williams's Obstetrics* p. 380. Norwalk, Connecticut: Appleton and Lange.

9 Albuquerque Journal, Monday July 6, 1992, page 1, Section B. Quoting study by researchers at the Jewish General Hospital and at McGill University in Montreal, Canada, published in the Online Journal of Current Clinical Trials.

CHAPTER 25: HOW TO GIVE BIRTH IF YOU NEED A CAESAREAN

1 Caldwell Sorel, Nancy (1984). *Ever Since Eve.* New York: Oxford University Press, pp. 109–110.

2 Ball, Aimee Lee (1993). The baby bust: Why more and more obstetricians are refusing to deliver. *New York Magazine,* January 25: 29–35.

3 Albers, Leah (Winter, 1994). Electronic fetal monitoring reassessed. *Child birth Instructor Magazine,* 24–27.

CHAPTER 27: GETTING DADS INVOLVED

Epigraph: Dass, Ram (1982). Preface to Levine, Stephen, *Who Dies.* p. vii. New York: Doubleday.

CHAPTER 28: PITFALLS OF LABOUR COACHING

1 Wagner, Marsden (1996). Audiotape of lecture: "Epidural epidemic." Midwifery Today Conference, Eugene, Oregon.

CHAPTER 30: THE FIRST MOMENTS

Epigraph on page 232: quote from Stevie Wonder from LIFE, 1986, p.71.

1 Dunham, Carroll and the Body Shop 'Ieam (1991). *Mamatoto: A celebration of birth* pp. 106–107. New York: Viking.

2 Hale, Christine (1991). Birth at home: An immanent power. *Mothering,* Spring:71–75.

CHAPTER 32: GATHERING INFORMATION

1 Schultz, Terry (1979). A nurse's view on circumcision. *Mothering* 26(XII), Summor Letter to the Editor.

INTRODUCTION TO SECTION VI (PAGE 190)

1 Goer, Henci (1995). *Obstetrical myths versus research realities: A guide to the medical literature* p. 252. Westport, Connecticut: Bergin & Garvey.

2 *Ibid* p. 252

CHAPTER 36: ECOLOGY OF PAIN

1 Brown, Christine (1982). Therapeutic effects of bathing during labor. *Journal of Nurse-Midwifery* vol. 27, No.1, Jan/Feb:13–16.

2 Dunham, Carroll and the Body Shop Team (1991). *Mamatoto: A cele-bration of birth* p. 90. New York: Viking.
3 Brown, Christine (1982). *op. cit.*
4 Erickson, Marlene (1994). Aromatherapy for childbearing. *Mothering*, Summer:75–79.
5 Dunham, Carroll. *op. cit.* p. 88.
6 Radin, Tari G. et al (1993). Nurses' care during labor: Its effect on the cesarean birth rate of healthy nulliparous women. *Birth* 20:1. March:14–20.

CHAPTER 37: DON'T GIVE BIRTH WITHOUT A DOULA
Epigraph, page 274: Perez, P. and Snedeker, C. (1990). *Special women: The role of the professional labor assistant* p. 105. Seattle, Washington: Pennypress, Inc.
Epigraph, page 278: *Ibid* p. 99.
1 Kennell, John, et al (1991). Continuous emotional support during labor in a US hospital: A randomized controlled trial. *JAMA.* May 1, 265(17):2197220 1.
2 Hofmeyer, GL et al (1991). Companionship to modify the clinical birth environment: Effects on progress and perceptions of labour and breast-feeding. *British Journal of Obstetrics and Gynecology* 98:756–764.
3 Wolman, WI., et al (May, 1993). Postpartum depression and compan-ionship in the clinical birth environment: A randomized controlled study. *American Journal of Obstetrics and Gynecology* 168(5):1388–1393.
4 Wolman, WI.. et al. *Ibid* pp. 1388–1393.
5 Klaus, Marshall, Kennell, John and Klaus, Phyllis (1993). *Mothering the mother*. Reading, MA: Addison Wesley.

CHAPTER 38: PROVEN PAIN TECHNIQUES
1 Heywood, Alison and Ho, Elaine (1990). Pain relief in labor. In Alexander, Jo, et al, Editors. *Intrapartum care* pp. 93–98.
2 Harrison, HF et al (1983). Pain relief in labor using transcutaneous electrical nerve stimulation (TEN.S). *British Journal of Obstetrics and Gynecology* 93:739–746.
3 Tawfik, et al (1982) cited in Heywood, Alison and Ho, Elaine *op. cit.* p. 98.
4 Heywood, Alison and Ho, Elaine (1990). *op. cit.* p. 95.

CHAPTER 39: THE COMPASSIONATE USE OF DRUGS AND EPIDURALS
1 Hannon, Sharron (1980). *Childbirth: A sourcebook for conception, preg-nancy, birth and the first weeks of life* p. 150. New York: M. Evans and Company, Inc.
2 Wagner, Marsden (1996). Audiotape of lecture: "Epidural epidemic" Midwifery Today Conference (1996) Eugene, Oregon.

3 Hale, Christine (1991). Birth at home: An immanent power. *Mothering*. Spring: 71–74.

4 Meigs, Dr. Charles quoted in Hannon, Sharron, *op. cit.*, p. 150.

5 Simkin, Penny (1996). Audiotape of lecture: "Epidural epidemic." Midwifery Today Conference, Oregon.

6 Wuitchik, Bakal and Lipshitz quoted in Goer, Henci (1995). Epidurals: Myths versus realities.Childbirth *Instructor Magazine* Winter: pp 17–20.

7 Thorp, James, et al. (1989). The effect of continuous epidural anesthesia on cesarean section for dystocia in nulliparous women. *American Journal of Obstetrics and Gynecologists*. 161(3), September:670–674.

8 Arms, Suzanne (1994). *Immaculate deception II: A fresh look at childbirth* p. 98. Berkeley, California: Celestial Arts.
Epigraph on page 325, Marsden Wagner, MD, from audiotape "Epidural epidemic" (co-presented with Penny Simkin). Midwifery Today Conference (1996), Eugene, Oregon.

9 Lagercrantz, H and Slotkin, T (1986). The Stress of Being Born. *Scientific American*. 254(4):100–107.

10 Goer, Henci (1995). *op. cit.*.

11 Murray, Ann D, et al (1981). Effects of epidural anesthesia on newborns and their mothers. *Child Development*. 52:71–82.

12 Ploekinger, Barbara, et al (1995). Epidural anaesthesia in labour: influence on surgical delivery rates, intrapartum fever and blood loss. *Gynecol Obstetrics Investigator*.39:24–27. and Avard, Denise M. and Nimrod, Carl M. (1985). Risks and benefits of obstetric analgesia: A review. *Birth*. 12(4), Winter:2 1 5–225.

13 Ramin, SM, et al (1995). Randomized trial of epidural versus intravenous analgesia during labor. *Obstetrics Gynecology*. 86:783–789.

14 Thorp, James, et al (1993). The effect of intrapartum epidural anesthesia on nulliparous labor: A randomized, controlled, prospective trial. *American Journal of Obstetrics and Gynecology* 169:4, Oct:851–858.

15 Thorp, James, et al (1993). *Ibid*.

16 Fusi, Luca, et al. (1989). Maternal pyrexia associated with the use of epidural anesalgesia in labour. *The Lancet*. June 3:1250–1252.

17 Macaulay, Bond, and Steer cited in Goer, Henci (1995) *op. cit.*

18 Fusi, Luca et al (1989). *op. cit.*

19 Fusi, Luca, et al (1989). *Ibid*.

20 Fusi, Luca, et al (1989), *Ibid*.

21 Abbound, TK, et al (1984). Continuous infusion epidural analgesia in parturients receiving bupivacaine, chloroprocaine, or lidocaine—maternal, fetal and newborn effects. *Anesthesia Anal*. 63:421–428.

22 Murray, Ann D. et al. *op.cit.*

23 Poore, Marta and Foster, Joyce Cameron (1985). Epidural and no epidural anesthesia: Differences between mothers and their experiences of birth. *Birth*, vol 12:4, Winter: 205–212.

Epigraph on page 329: Penny Simkin, PT, from audiotape "Epidural epidemic," a lecture co-presented at the Midwifery Today Conference (1996) Eugene, Oregon.

24 Simkin, Penny. Audiotape *op. cit.*
25 Simkin, Penny Audiotape *Ibid.*

Epigraph on page 330: Doris Haire, from lecture presented at *Midwifery Today Conference* (1996).

CHAPTER 40: GESTATING MOTHERHOOD

Epigraph: "Premature": Webster's New Twentieth Century Dictionary, Second Edition, 1983, NewYork: Simon and Schuster.

CHAPTER 41: BABY-PROOFING YOUR MARRIAGE

1 Belsky, Jay and Kelly, John (1994). *The transition to parenthood: How a first child changes a marriage* p. 13. New York: Delacorte Press.
2 *Ibid*, p. 14–15.
3 *Ibid*, p. 33.
4 *Ibid*, p. 16.
5 *Ibid*, p. 32.
6 Leigh, Dominique (1990). Zen dust, zen sweep. *Mothering* Winter:28–30.

CHAPTER 42 SWADDLING THE NEW PARENTS

Epigraphs on page 348: Goldsmith, Judith (1984). *Childbirth wisdom: From the world's oldest societies* p. 69, 86. New York: Congdon & Weed, Inc.

1 Arms, Suzanne (1994). *Immaculate Deception II: A fresh look at childbirth* p. 195. Berkeley, California: Celestial Arts.
2 Korte, Diana and Scaer, Roberta (1984). *A good birth, a safe birth* p. 11. Toronto: Bantam Books.
3 Brook, Danae (1976). *Naturebirth* p. 237. London: Heinemann.
4 Arms, Suzanne, *op. cit.* p. 201.

APPENDIX B

1 Healthy Parenting. *Prevention.* March 1996:42 referring to Mehl, Lewis E. (1994). *Archives of Family Medicine* vol 3.

APPENDIX E

1 Wiener, Rosemary (1980). Circumcision. *Mothering* Summer: 35–39.

INDEX

ABOUT THE AUTHORS

PAM ENGLAND, C. N. M., M. A.

As a midwife and mother, Pam realized the chasm between what was being offered in traditional childbirth classes and what women were needing to prepare to give birth. In 1989, Pam began creating the Birthing From Within approach to help mothers reclaim the spiritual, emotional, and psychological awareness needed to fully experience birth as the rite of passage it is and should be.

Pam is a registered nurse, and received her midwifery training from the Frontier Nursing Service, Hyden, Kentucky. She has sixteen years experience attending births in hospital, home, and birth center. Later, Pam earned a master's degree from Antioch University in psychology and counseling, specializing in prenatal-birth and postpartum therapy. Her thesis was a study of Childbirth Images of Modern and Ancient Women.

Pam developed and directs the Art of Birthing Doula Training Program, and in 1995, founded the Art of Birthing Center in Albuquerque. She enjoys mothering her two sons, making Ikebana (Japanese flower arrangements), and drawing and painting.

ROB HOROWITZ, PH. D.

Rob grew up in New York City where he attended the Bronx High School of Science. After receiving his bachelor's degree in English Literature from the University of Rochester, he taught English for four years in an inner-city Bronx high school. He wandered around Europe, then returned to the U.S. and earned master's and doctoral degrees in clinical psychology from Peabody College of Vanderbilt University (1981). He did his clinical psychology residency at the Department of Psychiatry, University of Texas Medical Branch (Galveston), where he specialized in family therapy and systems interventions.

He loves fathering, and enjoys gardening, backpacking with buddies in the Wyoming wilderness, and playing tournament bridge with his bright-eyed 101-year-old dad, Norman. Yoga and golf help him maintain appropriate levels of humility, as well as offering additional opportunities to continue exploring coping with physical and mental pain. He maintains a private therapy practice in Albuquerque.

"The Bible of baby massage … crammed full of information and pictures demonstrating how your healing hands can help your baby." *'Junior'*

Infant Massage
Vimala McClure

£9.99

Master the techniques of infant massage so that you incorporate this wonderful healing art into your baby's life. Vimala McClure shows how a daily massage can be one of the greatest gifts a child can receive, bringing physical and psychological benefits to both parents and babies.

Massage benefits babies – easing discomfort; releasing tension; helping premature babies to gain weight; relief of colic, fever, chest and nasal congestion – as well as bonding the baby to its parents.

"What was available before, when I was a nervous first time mum? How I wish I had been aware of the gentle teachings of Vimala McClure … This woman talks my kind of language – that touch is such a powerful communicator." *'Positive Health'*

"This is the man who has made childbirth a delightful,
natural experience for so many women."
'*Nursery World*'

Birth Reborn
Michel Odent

£12.99

For over 40 years Michel Odent has been the world's leading 'birth guru'. He has pioneered a new philosophy of childbirth, making it a natural experience for women and providing settings that allow a woman to give birth her own way. Women become their own birthing experts, if they follow their instincts they can birth naturally, with the minimal intervention of medical science.

Birth Reborn gives expectant mothers the confidence and information they need in order to trust themselves to give birth without the drugs and medical procedures that are being increasingly recognised as harmful to the mother and to the baby's future development.

"Combining the roles of romantic, philosopher, surgeon
and obstetrician as only a Frenchman could ... many of
(Michel Odent's) theories have changed the way
childbirth is viewed and conducted."
'*The Times*'

This lively, highly readable little book is for everyone who works with maternity and neonatal services ... a heartening, honest, practical, non-nonsense guide to a method of care that will appeal to most people for sensible reasons."
'*Infant Journal*'

Kangaroo Babies
Nathalie Charpak

£14.99

Kangaroo Mother Care was created to help premature and low-birth-weight-infants develop into healthy babies. The baby remains in direct skin-to-skin contact with its mother who provides, naturally, all the benefits of incubator care: the baby's body temperature is regulated, breastfeeding is stimulated, bonding is strengthened and the baby feels secure.

It is a natural approach to mothering, which will revolutionise the care of all newborn babies.

"We needed the well-documented book by Nathalie Charpak – an active member of the Kangaroo Foundation – to realize that the concept of marsupial babies is spreading at a high speed all over the world."
Michel Odent, author of 'Birth Reborn'